D1263733

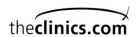

CLINICS IN SPORTS MEDICINE

ACL Graft and Fixation Choices

GUEST EDITORS
Jon K. Sekiya, MD
Steven B. Cohen, MD

CONSULTING EDITOR
Mark D. Miller, MD

October 2007 • Volume 26 • Number 4

SAUNDERS
An Imprint of Elsevier, Inc.
PHILADELPHIA   LONDON   TORONTO   MONTREAL   SYDNEY   TOKYO

W.B. SAUNDERS COMPANY
A Division of Elsevier Inc.

1600 John F. Kennedy Blvd. • Suite 1800 • Philadelphia, Pennsylvania 19103

http://www.theclinics.com

CLINICS IN SPORTS MEDICINE	**Volume 26, Number 4**
October 2007	**ISSN 0278-5919**
Editor: Debora Dellapena	**ISBN-13: 978-1-4160-5057-5**
	ISBN-10: 1-4160-5057-4

The ideas and opinions expressed in *Clinics in Sports Medicine* do not necessarily reflect those of the Publisher. The Publisher does not assume any responsibility for any injury and/or damage to persons or property arising out of or related to any use of the material contained in this periodical. The reader is advised to check the appropriate medical literature and the product information currently provided by the manufacturer of each drug to be administered to verify the dosage, the method and duration of administration, or contraindications. It is the responsibility of the treating physician or other health care professional, relying on independent experience and knowledge of the patient, to determine drug dosages and the best treatment for the patient. Mention of any product in this issue should not be construed as endorsement by the contributors, editors, or the Publisher of the product or manufacturers' claims.

Clinics in Sports Medicine (ISSN 0278-5919) is published quarterly by Elsevier Inc., 360 Park Avenue South, New York, NY 10010-1710. Months of publication are January, April, July, and October. Business and Editorial Offices: 1600 John F. Kennedy Blvd., Suite 1800, Philadelphia, PA 19103-2899. Customer Service Offices: 6277 Sea Harbor Drive, Orlando, FL 32887-4800. Periodicals postage paid at New York, NY, and additional mailing offices. Subscription prices are $205.00 per year (US individuals), $313.00 per year (US institutions), $103.00 per year (US students), $232.00 per year (Canadian individuals), $371.00 per year (Canadian institutions), $135.00 (Canadian students), $265.00 per year (foreign individuals), $371.00 per year (foreign institutions), and $135.00 per year (foreign students). Foreign air speed delivery is included in all *Clinics* subscription prices. All prices are subject to change without notice. POSTMASTER: Send address changes to *Clinics in Sports Medicine*, Elsevier Periodicals Customer Service, 6277 Sea Harbor Drive, Orlando, FL 32887-4800. **Customer Service: 1-800-654-2452 (US). From outside of the US, call 1-407-345-4000.** E-mail: hhspcs@harcourt.com.

Clinics in Sports Medicine is covered in *Index Medicus, Current Contents/Clinical Medicine, Excerpta Medica,* and *ISI/Biomed.*

Printed in the United States of America.

ELSEVIER
SAUNDERS

CLINICS IN SPORTS MEDICINE

ACL Graft and Fixation Choices

CONSULTING EDITOR

MARK D. MILLER, MD, Professor, Department of Orthopaedic Surgery; and Head, Division of Sports Medicine, University of Virginia Health Systems, Charlottesville, Virginia

GUEST EDITORS

JON K. SEKIYA, MD, Associate Professor, MedSport, Department of Orthopaedic Surgery; and Team Physician, University of Michigan, Ann Arbor, Michigan

STEVEN B. COHEN, MD, Director of Sports Medicine Research, Rothman Institute Orthopaedics; Assistant Professor, Department of Orthopaedic Surgery, Thomas Jefferson University, Philadelphia, Pennsylvania

CONTRIBUTORS

BERNARD R. BACH, Jr, MD, Professor and Director, Division of Sports Medicine, Rush University Medical Center, Chicago, Illinois

GEOFFREY S. BAER, MD, PhD, Sports Medicine Fellow, Department of Orthopaedic Surgery, University of Pittsburgh Medical Center, Pittsburgh, Pennsylvania

JEFF C. BRAND, Jr, MD, Alexandria Orthopaedics and Sports Medicine Asssociates, Alexandria, Minnesota

CHARLES H. BROWN, Jr, MD, Medical Director, Abu Dhabi Knee and Sports Medicine Centre, Abu Dhabi, United Arab Emirates

MATTHEW L. BUSAM, MD, Surgeon, Cincinnati Sports Medicine Research and Education, Foundation, Cincinnati, Ohio

NEAL C. CHEN, MD, Orthopaedic Resident, Combined Harvard Orthopaedic Residency Program; Clinical Fellow, Hand and Upper Extremity Service, Massachusetts General Hospital, Boston, Massachusetts; Clinical Fellow, Sports Medicine and Shoulder Service, Hospital for Special Surgery, New York, New York

STEVEN B. COHEN, MD, Director of Sports Medicine Research, Rothman Institute Orthopaedics; Assistant Professor, Department of Orthopaedic Surgery, Thomas Jefferson University, Philadelphia, Pennsylvania

JOSEPH P. DeANGELIS, MD, Resident, Department of Orthopaedic Surgery, University of Connecticut School of Medicine, Farmington, Connecticut

MICHAEL J. ELLIOTT, MD, Director of Orthopedics, Department of Orthopedics, Specialty Medical Group, Children's Hospital Central California, Madera, California; and Assistant Professor of Surgery, Department of Orthopedics Uniformed Services University of the Health Sciences, Bethesda, Maryland

CRISTIN M. FERGUSON, MD, Department of Orthopaedic Surgery, Wake Forest University School of Medicine, Winston-Salem, North Carolina

FREDDIE H. FU, MD, DSc(Hon), DPs(Hon), Professor and Chairman, Department of Orthopaedic Surgery, University of Pittsburgh, Pittsburgh, Pennsylvania

JOHN P. FULKERSON, MD, Clinical Professor and Sports Medicine Fellowship Director, Department of Orthopaedic Surgery, University of Connecticut School of Medicine; Orthopedic Associates of Hartford, P.C., Farmington, Connecticut

TINKER GRAY, MA, Research Director, Shelbourne Knee Center at Methodist Hospital, Indianapolis, Indiana

LAWRENCE V. GULOTTA, MD, Resident, Department of Orthopaedic Surgery, Hospital for Special Surgery, Weill Medical College of Cornell University, New York, New York

CHRISTOPHER D. HARNER, MD, Medical Director, Center for Sports Medicine; and Professor, Department of Orthopaedic Surgery, University of Pittsburgh Medical Center, Pittsburgh, Pennsylvania

STEPHEN M. HOWELL, MD, Associate Professor, Department of Mechanical and Aeronautical Engineering, University of California Davis, Davis, California

CHRISTOPHER A. KURTZ, MD, Assistant Professor of Surgery, Department of Orthopedics, Uniformed Services University of the Health Sciences; and Head, Division of Sports Medicine Department of Orthopaedic Surgery, Naval Medical Center Portsmouth, Portsmouth Virginia

KEITH W. LAWHORN, MD, Assistant Professor of Surgery, Uniformed Services University of the Health Sciences, Bethesda, Maryland; and Advanced Orthopaedics and Sports Medicine Institute, Fairfax, Virginia

MAHIR MAHIROGULLARI, MD, Department of Orthopaedic Surgery, Gulhane Medical Faculty, GATA Haydarpasa Training Hospital, Uskudar Istanbul, Turkey; Department of Orthopaedic Surgery, Wake Forest University School of Medicine, Winston-Salem, North Carolina

MARK D. MILLER, MD, Professor, Department of Orthopaedic Surgery; and Head, Division of Sports Medicine, University of Virginia Health Systems, Charlottesville, Virginia

GARY G. POEHLING, MD, Department of Orthopaedic Surgery, Wake Forest University School of Medicine, Winston-Salem, North Carolina

SCOTT A. RODEO, MD, Associate Attending Orthopaedic Surgeon, Hospital for Special Surgery; Associate Professor of Orthopaedic Surgery, Weill Medical College of Cornell University, New York, New York

JOHN-PAUL H. RUE, MD, LCDR, MC, USN, Department of Orthopaedics, National Naval Medical Center, Bethesda, Maryland

ROBERT J. SCHODERBEK, Jr, MD, Orthopaedic Resident, Department of Orthopaedic Surgery, University of Virginia Health Systems, Charlottesville, Virginia

JON K. SEKIYA, MD, Associate Professor, MedSport, Department of Orthopaedic Surgery; and Team Physician, University of Michigan, Ann Arbor, Michigan

K. DONALD SHELBOURNE, MD, Orthopaedic Surgeon, Shelbourne Knee Center at Methodist Hospital; Associate Clinical Professor, Indiana University School of Medicine, Indianapolis, Indiana

WEI SHEN, MD, PhD, Postdoctoral Research Associate, Department of Orthopaedic Surgery, University of Pittsburgh, Pittsburgh, Pennsylvania

KATHRYNE J. STABILE, MD, MS, Department of Orthopaedic Surgery, Wake Forest University School of Medicine, Winston-Salem, North Carolina

SAMIR G. TEJWANI, MD, Associate, Kaiser Permanente, Department of Orthopaedic Surgery, Fontana, California

GEHRON P. TREME, MD, Orthopadic Sports Medicine Fellow, Department of Orthopaedic Surgery, University of Virginia Health Systems, Charlottesville, Virginia

BAVORNRAT VANADURONGWAN, MD, Research Fellow, Shelbourne Knee Center at Methodist Hospital, Indianapolis, Indiana

PATRICK W. WHITLOCK, MD, PhD, Department of Orthopaedic Surgery, Wake Forest University School of Medicine, Winston-Salem, North Carolina

CLINICS IN SPORTS MEDICINE

ELSEVIER
SAUNDERS

ACL Graft and Fixation Choices

CONTENTS
VOLUME 26 • NUMBER 4 • OCTOBER 2007

The graft-bone attachment site is the weak link in anterior cruciate ligament (ACL) reconstruction surgery because healing is slow and often incomplete. Each of the many graft options for ACL reconstruction surgery has different healing characteristics and potential. Autografts that allow bone-to-bone healing offer the best healing potential. An understanding of the biology of graft healing should give the surgeon context in graft selection and rehabilitation for ACL reconstruction.

The anterior cruciate ligament (ACL) serves an important stabilizing and biomechanical function for the knee. Reconstruction of the ACL remains one of the most commonly performed procedures in the field of sports medicine. Reconstruction of the ACL with bone-patella tendon-bone (BPTB) autograft secured with interference screw fixation has been the historical reference standard and remains the benchmark against which other methods are gauged. This article reviews the reconstruction of the ACL with BPTB autograft including the surgical technique, rationale for BTPB use, and outcomes.

Primary ACL reconstruction using a contralateral patellar tendon autograft is an effective means of achieving symmetrical range of motion and strength after surgery. When the graft is harvested from the ipsilateral knee, the rehabilitation for the ACL graft and for the graft-donor site are different and have opposing goals. Rehabilitation for the ACL graft involves obtaining full range of motion, reducing swelling, and providing the appropriate stress to achieve graft maturation. Rehabilitation for the graft-donor site involves performing high-repetition strengthening exercises to regain size and strength, best achieved when begun immediately after surgery.

The use of autogenous hamstring tendon as a graft source for anterior cruciate ligament (ACL) reconstruction continues to gain in popularity. The low harvest morbidity and excellent biomechanical graft properties coupled with improved fixation of soft tissue grafts are all reasons for excellent clinical outcomes of ACL reconstruction using hamstring tendons. In addition, surgeon awareness of the complications associated with poor tunnel placement and more exacting tunnel placement techniques help prevent roof and posterior cruciate ligament impingement and contribute to the successful outcomes of hamstring ACL constructs.

Anterior cruciate ligament (ACL) reconstruction surgery with the central third quadriceps tendon can yield a stable, high-functioning knee with little associated morbidity. Both the quadriceps tendon-patellar bone graft and the free tendon graft are reported to produce good to excellent outcomes at more than 2 years of follow-up. The decreased donor-site morbidity and absence of anterior knee pain suggest that the quadriceps free tendon autograft offers a reliable, pain-free, low-morbidity autograft alternative in ACL reconstruction. Recent data suggest that this graft may be the least morbid of the currently used ACL autograft reconstruction alternatives.

Allograft tissue seems to provide an excellent option for reconstruction of the ACL in the primary and revision setting. Although in general the risks of using allograft tissue in ACL reconstruction are low, the consequences of complications associated with disease or infection transmission or of recurrent instability secondary to graft failure are large. Surgeons should provide patients with the information available regarding allograft risks and should have thorough knowledge of the source and preparation of the grafts by their tissue bank before implantation for ACL reconstruction.

Reconstruction of the anterior cruciate ligament provides consistently good to excellent results allowing return to work and sport. Allograft tissue is an alternative to autografts when appropriate donor tissue is not available or its use is not advisable for other reasons. The technique and results for allograft use are similar to those for autograft, making its use appropriate in a variety of clinical scenarios. This article reviews the indications for allograft ACL reconstruction, graft options, and technique for allograft use.

Freeze-dried allografts represent a viable and functional alternative to fresh-frozen allograft and autograft constructs. Compared with fresh-frozen allograft constructs, freeze-dried soft tissue allograft constructs have many advantages including limited immunogenicity, ease of graft storage, comparable mechanical properties of soft tissue constructs, and the potential for improved biologic incorporation. This article reviews the fundamental processing of freeze-dried allografts and summarizes the clinical and basic science studies supporting the safe and effective use of freeze-dried allograft constructs for anterior cruciate ligament reconstruction. It also discusses potential directions of future research on tissue-engineered anterior cruciate ligament constructs using freeze-dried tendon constructs.

The anterior cruciate ligament (ACL) is composed of two functional bundles, the anteromedial and posterolateral. Multiple biomechanical and clinical studies have demonstrated that the posterolateral bundle plays a critical role in rotatory stability of the knee. Anatomic double-bundle reconstruction of the ACL best restores knee function and kinematics when the ACL is ruptured. For double-bundle ACL reconstruction, the use of allograft is safe, minimizes graft harvest morbidity, expedites recovery, and is associated with successful clinical results in short-term follow-up.

Anterior cruciate ligament (ACL) injuries are the most common complete ligamentous injury to the knee. The optimal graft should be able to reproduce the anatomy and biomechanics of the ACL, be incorporated rapidly with strong initial fixation, and cause low graft-site morbidity. This article reviews the literature comparing the clinical outcomes following allograft and autograft ACL reconstruction and examines current issues regarding graft choice.

ELSEVIER
SAUNDERS

CLINICS IN SPORTS MEDICINE

Clin Sports Med 26 (2007) xiii

CLINICS IN SPORTS MEDICINE

ELSEVIER
SAUNDERS

Foreword

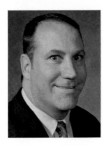

Mark D. Miller, MD

Consulting Editor

ACL reconstruction has been such a popular topic that many journals have made an effort not to publish new papers on this subject over the past several years. Nevertheless, this subject has thrust itself back into the limelight and has been the subject of much recent controversy and debate. How can an operative procedure that has been one of our most successful surgeries over the years possibly be modified and improved upon? The answer appears to be that we must be more critical with ourselves regarding what is considered to be a "success." The pivotal issue appears to be eliminating the pivot shift rotational instability for the lifetime of the knee.

This issue of *Clinics in Sports Medicine* focuses on new research into anterior cruciate ligament (ACL) grafts, fixation, and other important aspects of ACL reconstruction. Drs. Sekiya and Cohen, like myself, are both graduates of the University of Pittsburgh Sports Medicine Fellowship program, the home of the double-bundle ACL. I must note that they showed amazing constraint in not including an article on that subject. Perhaps that could serve as a stand-alone topic for a future issue of *Clinics in Sports Medicine*. I hope you enjoy this outstanding issue.

Mark D. Miller, MD
Department of Orthopedic Surgery
Division of Sports Medicine
University of Virginia Health System
P.O. Box 800753
Charlottesville, VA 22903-0753, USA

E-mail address: MDM3P@hscmail.mcc.virginia.edu

0278-5919/07/$ – see front matter
doi:10.1016/j.csm.2007.07.001

Clin Sports Med 26 (2007) xv–xvi

CLINICS IN SPORTS MEDICINE

Preface

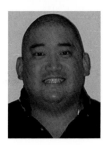
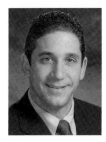

Jon K. Sekiya, MD
Steven B. Cohen, MD

Guest Editors

The need for reconstruction of the torn anterior cruciate ligament (ACL) in the active patient is not controversial. There are, however, many other aspects of ACL reconstruction that are widely debated. Examples of the topics under discussion include type of graft, single or double bundle, type of fixation, and graft healing.

This issue of *Clinics in Sports Medicine* reviews some of the most common topics of discussion for surgeons performing ACL reconstruction. Specifically, this issue reviews the variety of grafts most commonly used. The type of graft used in ACL reconstruction is generally based on surgeon preference and comfort. Some surgeons prefer only allograft or autograft, whereas others select a graft based on the individual patient. The gold standard of bone-patellar tendon-bone (BPTB) autograft has given way, over recent years, to a selection of autografts, including hamstring (semitendinosis/gracilus), quadriceps tendon, and contralateral BPTB. All of these grafts have shown excellent results, with improvement in function and stability. In opposition, allograft use in recent years has steadily increased. Owing to increased availability, low donor site morbidity, decreased surgical time, improved preparation and safety, and decreased postoperative pain, allografts have gained popularity. Yet, there is still debate on type of allograft (soft tissue, Achilles tendon, and BPTB) and preparation (fresh-frozen or freeze-dried). Regardless of type of graft or its preparation, the outcome results of allograft reconstruction appear to be comparable to those of autograft reconstruction.

Of course, one of the hottest topics in ACL surgery is single- or double-bundle reconstruction. Freddie Fu, one of the pioneers of double-bundle reconstruction in North America, reviews the concepts and techniques in this

0278-5919/07/$ – see front matter
doi:10.1016/j.csm.2007.06.012

issue. Additional chapters are dedicated to allograft safety and the biology of graft healing. Finally, the issues of specific fixation with regard to aperture and peripheral fixation, and the biomechanics of graft fixation, are reviewed in great detail.

The authors of the chapters in this issue should be commended for their thorough and timely contributions. All are experts in the field of ACL surgery. We would like to thank Mark D. Miller, MD, one of our mentors, for the opportunity to contribute to this edition of *Clinics in Sports Medicine*. In addition, we would like to thank Deb Dellapena of Elsevier for her assistance in the preparation of this edition.

Jon K. Sekiya, MD
MedSport, Department of Orthopaedic Surgery
University of Michigan
24 Frank Lloyd Wright Drive, PO Box 0391
Ann Arbor, MI 48106, USA

E-mail address: sekiya@med.umich.edu

Steven B. Cohen, MD
Department of Orthopaedic Surgery
Thomas Jefferson University
Rothman Institute of Orthopaedics
925 Chestnut Street
Philadelphia, PA 19107, USA

E-mail address: steven.cohen@rothmaninstitute.com

Clin Sports Med 26 (2007) 509–524

CLINICS IN SPORTS MEDICINE

ELSEVIER
SAUNDERS

Biology of Autograft and Allograft Healing in Anterior Cruciate Ligament Reconstruction

Lawrence V. Gulotta, MD, Scott A. Rodeo, MD*

Hospital for Special Surgery, Weill Medical College of Cornell University, 535 E. 70th Street, New York, NY 10021, USA

Operative reconstruction of a torn or insufficient anterior cruciate ligament (ACL) has become a routine surgical procedure in orthopedics. The most commonly used grafts for this procedure are autologous bone-patellar tendon-bone, hamstring, and quadriceps tendons. Allografts in the form of Achilles tendons, bone-patellar tendon-bone, hamstring tendon, fascia lata, tibialis anterior tendon, and posterior tibialis tendon also are gaining popularity. Biomechanical testing has shown that the initial strength of these graft materials is higher than that of the intact ACL [1,2]. Therefore, the weakest link following reconstruction is not the graft itself but rather the femoral and tibial fixation points [3]. This realization has led to the development of several commercially available fixation devices for graft fixation. All orthopaedic fixation devices, however, are merely temporizing components until tissue healing occurs. Ultimately, the long-term success of an ACL reconstruction depends on the ability of the graft to heal adequately in a bone tunnel. The intra-articular portion of the graft also must undergo the process of ligamentization in which the tendon graft remodels to form a structure similar to a normal ligament. An understanding of the biology of graft healing in the bone tunnel and graft intra-articular remodeling is critical for surgeons to make appropriate graft choices for their patients.

The principal form of healing that occurs in the bone tunnel depends on the graft used. Autologous bone-patellar tendon-bone offers the strongest healing potential because it relies mainly on bone-to-bone healing between the graft bone plug and the tunnel [4,5]. Even with bone-patellar tendon-bone grafts, there is some component of tendon-to-bone healing because some of the tendinous portion of the graft usually remains at the tunnel aperture (opening into the joint). Although bone-patellar tendon-bone grafts remain very popular, concerns about donor-site morbidity have caused some surgeons to search for alternative graft sources.

*Corresponding author. *E-mail address*: RodeoS@HSS.EDU (S.A. Rodeo).

0278-5919/07/$ – see front matter
doi:10.1016/j.csm.2007.06.007

Autologous hamstring grafts have less donor-site morbidity but rely solely on the tendon-to-bone healing. This process occurs slowly and never recapitulates the native ACL insertion site in morphology or in mechanical strength, leading to concerns about graft pullout and slippage resulting in instability and eventual failure. Allografts obviate the need for a donor site and therefore have no associated donor-site morbidity. Although the use of these grafts is growing in popularity, concerns remain regarding disease transmission, infection, tunnel widening caused by immune response, and delayed healing.

Because all grafts depend on some degree on tendon-to-bone healing, this article focuses mainly on the current understanding of how this process takes place and discusses strategies to improve healing. The biology of bone-to-bone healing of a graft, the process of intra-articular graft remodeling, and the specific characteristics of allograft healing also are discussed.

TENDON-TO-BONE HEALING IN ANTERIOR CRUCIATE LIGAMENT RECONSTRUCTION

The normal tendon or ligament insertion into bone is a highly specialized tissue that functions to transmit complex mechanical loads from soft tissue to bone. Ligaments have two distinct types of insertion sites: direct and indirect. The ACL inserts into the bone through a direct insertion site that transitions from tendon to bone (**Fig. 1**). This transition contains four distinct zones: tendon, unmineralized fibrocartilage, mineralized fibrocartilage, and bone. Cartilage-specific collagens including types II, IX, X, and XI are found in the fibrocartilage of the insertion site with collagen X playing a fundamental role in maintaining the interface between mineralized and unmineralized

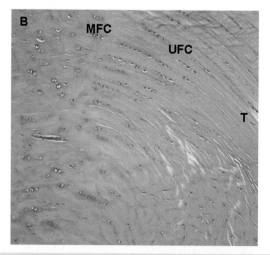

Fig. 1. Normal tendon-to-bone direct insertion site of the rabbit ACL. Note the four zones: tendon (T), unmineralized fibrocartilage (UFC), mineralized fibrocartilage (MFC), and bone (B).

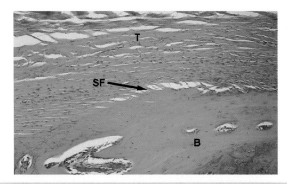

Fig. 2. Normal tendon-to-bone indirect insertion site of the rabbit MCL with Sharpey's fibers. B, bone; SF, Sharpey's fibers; T, tendon .

fibrocartilage [6–8]. This composition is in contrast to ligaments like the medial collateral ligament of the knee that insert into bone through an indirect insertion site (Fig. 2). Indirect insertion sites are composed of collagen fibers called Sharpey's fibers that are directed obliquely to the long axis of the bone. These fibers anchor the ligament into bone and confer mechanical strength.

The structure and composition of the normal ACL direct insertion site is not reproduced after ligament reconstruction with tendon grafts. Studies have shown that instead of regenerating the four zones of the native direct insertion site, the graft heals with an interposed layer of fibrovascular scar tissue at the graft–tunnel interface (Fig. 3) [9–11]. By 3 to 4 weeks after surgery, the collagen at this interface organizes and forms perpendicular fibers resembling the Sharpey's fibers of an indirect attachment site (Fig. 4) [10,11]. These fibers continue to be present 1 year after surgery, and their number and size are positively

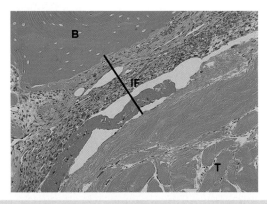

Fig. 3. Tendon-to-bone interface after ACL reconstruction with a tendon graft in a rabbit at 1 week. Note the fibrovascular interface (scar) tissue between the tendon and the bone. B, bone; IF, interface tissue; T, tendon.

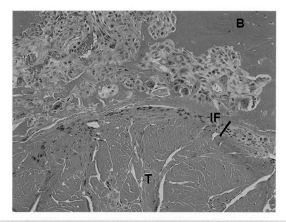

Fig. 4. Tendon-to-bone interface at 2 weeks. Note the decrease in interface tissue at 2 weeks. B, bone; IF, interface tissue; T, tendon.

correlated with the pull-out strength of the graft (Fig. 5) [9–11]. Eventually bone grows into the interface tissue and incorporates the outer portion of the graft, improving graft attachment strength [11].

Kanazawa and colleagues [12] used immunohistochemistry to examine the maturing process of tendon grafts in the bone tunnel of a rabbit ACL reconstruction model. They found that in the initial postoperative period, the graft–tunnel interface is filled with granulation tissue containing type III collagen. Vascular endothelial growth factor (VEGF) and basic fibroblast growth

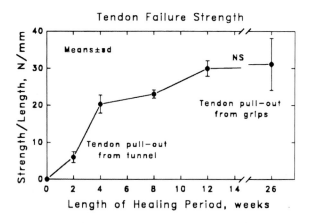

Fig. 5. Normalized values for interface strength plotted against healing time in a dog model. There are significant differences between each time-period until 12 weeks. NS, not significant (*From* Rodeo SA, Arnoczky SP, Torzilli PA, et al. Tendon-healing in a bone tunnel. A biomechanical and histological study in the dog. J Bone Joint Surg [Am] 1993;75(12):1802; with permission.)

factor are expressed, resulting in migration of enlarged fibroblasts, vascular endothelia, and macrophages. Chondroid cells that are S-100–positive then appear from the side of the bone tunnel and begin to degrade the granulation tissue and deposit type II collagen. The degradation of the granulation tissue stops short of the graft, and the number of S-100–positive chondroid cells decreases as the tissue is replaced by maturing lamellar bone. These histologic changes at the wall of the bone tunnel are similar to the process of endochondral ossification, with the environment of the bone tunnel similar to that of a fracture [13]. Finally, Sharpey's-like fibers appear that are composed of type III collagen and are oriented in a direction to counteract shear stresses. During this process, the tendinous graft initially becomes hypocellular. Then basic fibroblast growth factor is expressed from the margins of the tendon that signals the migration of spindle-shaped fibroblasts from the bone tunnel into the graft that then produce type III collagen. The authors noted that this process took approximately 8 weeks [12].

Because tendon-to-bone healing in ACL reconstructions with tendon grafts is inefficient, several studies have investigated ways to help augment and improve healing. Increasing the graft contact with the surrounding bone in the tunnel helps improve healing. Studies have shown that increasing the length of the bone tunnel positively correlates with the quality and strength of the reconstruction [14]. Minimizing the mismatch of graft and tunnel diameters, thereby tightening the fit of the graft in the tunnel, also improves healing [15]. Likewise, allowing circumferential contact between the graft and the tunnel (ie, no interference screw) also can improve healing [16]. Although it is clear that graft contact with the bone tunnel is important for healing, it is likely that more substantial improvements in tendon-to-bone healing will come from manipulation of the biologic environment at the healing tendon-bone interface.

The biology of healing between grafted tendons and bone remains incompletely understood. Current work suggests that several fundamental factors are responsible for the ineffective healing response between tendon and bone: (1) the presence of inflammation at the graft site that results in scar formation; (2) slow or limited bone ingrowth into the tendon graft, which results in a weaker attachment; (3) graft-tunnel motion that promotes the formation of granulation tissue rather than firm attachments; (4) an insufficient number of undifferentiated progenitor cells at the healing tendon–bone interface; and (5) lack of a coordinated signaling cascade that directs healing toward regeneration as opposed to scar tissue formation.

The earliest cellular response following surgical implantation of a tendon graft in a bone tunnel involves the accumulation of inflammatory cells. Kawamura and colleagues [17] evaluated the cells responsible for the early inflammatory response in a rodent ACL reconstruction model. They found that two distinct subpopulations of macrophages are present at the healing interface: the proinflammatory ED1+ macrophages and the proregenerative ED2+ macrophages. The ED1+ macrophages are derived from the circulation and, in conjunction with neutrophils, release cytokines such as transforming growth factor beta (TGF-β) that initiate the inflammatory response and promote scar formation. In a follow-up study, Hays and colleagues [18] found that tendon-to-bone healing occurs with less scar formation, more organized collagen deposition, and improved pull-out strengths when macrophages are depleted by administering intraperitoneal injections of liposomal clodronate (a bisphosphonate that selectively induces macrophage apoptosis).

Although macrophages seem to play a role in the production of a mechanically inferior scar interface, studies on other methods of reducing the immune response have produced conflicting results. The novel anti-inflammatory peptide, stable gastric pentadecapeptide BPC 157 (which is in trials for the treatment of inflammatory bowel disease), was found to improve Achilles tendon-to-bone healing in a rat model based on functional, biomechanical, and histologic criteria [19]. In this study, the ability of the Achilles tendon to heal to the enthesis was evaluated after resection; therefore healing in a bone tunnel was not evaluated. Cohen and colleagues [20], however, showed that administering the anti-inflammatory medications indomethacin and celecoxib, a selective cyclo-oxygenase 2 (COX-2) inhibitor, after rat supraspinatus repair actually delayed healing. The groups treated with either of the anti-inflammatory medications showed significantly decreased loads-to-failure at 2, 4, and 8 weeks, and the collagen was significantly more disorganized on polarized microscopy at 4 and 8 weeks than in controls. Although this study focused on a rotator cuff model rather than graft healing in a bone tunnel, these findings suggest the cyclo-oxygenase enzymes may be important in early tendon-to-bone healing. A recent study found that COX-2 plays a critical role in the incorporation of structural allografts, suggesting that cyclo-oxygenase may exert its positive effects in graft healing through new bone formation [21].

Bone ingrowth plays an important role in graft-to-bone healing because this stage of healing coincides with improved load-to-graft failures [11]. Several studies have investigated strategies to improve bone ingrowth into a tendon graft. Osteoinductive factors such as bone morphogenetic proteins (BMP) [22,23], osteoconductive agents such as calcium-phosphate cement, and osteoclast inhibition have been studied as potential strategies to improve bone formation around a tendon graft.

Rodeo and colleagues [23] delivered recombinant human BMP-2 (rhBMP-2) on an absorbable type I collagen sponge to a canine, extra-articular, tendon-to-bone healing model. At all time points, the rhBMP-2–treated limbs healed with more extensive bone formation around the tendon. Biomechanical testing demonstrated higher tendon pull-out strength in the rhBMP-2–treated side at 2 weeks. Experimenting with different carriers, Ma and colleagues [24] evaluated the use of rhBMP-2 in an injectable calcium phosphate matrix in an intra-articular model of rabbit ACL reconstruction. They also found that rhBMP-2 treatment led to a significant increase in the width of new bone formation and a decrease in the width of scar formation at the tendon–bone interface in a dose-dependent fashion. The rhBMP-2 group also demonstrated significantly increased stiffness at 8 weeks. Martinek and colleagues [25] used

hormone family such as insulin growth factor-1 and platelet-derived growth factor may improve tendon-to-bone healing based on histologic and biomechanical testing [35–39].

Vascularity is critical for efficient connective tissue healing; however, it is unclear if strategies to increase local vascularity at the tendon graft attachment can improve healing. Krivic [19] showed that stable gastric pentadecapeptide BPC 157 improved vascularity in an Achilles tendon-to-bone healing model and that this improved vascularity resulted in improved histologic and biomechanical properties. In contrast, a recent study examined the effect of VEGF, which is a potent mediator of angiogenesis, on graft healing in a sheep ACL reconstruction model [40]. In the experimental group, the grafts were soaked in VEGF. In the control group, the grafts were soaked in phosphate buffered saline. Although there was increased vascularity in the VEGF-treated group, the stiffness of the femur-graft-tibia complex in the VEGF-treated group was significantly lower than in controls. Although only a single concentration of VEGF solution was used, and the animals were evaluated at only one time point (12 weeks), these preliminary data suggest that excessive vascularity may have detrimental effects on the healing ACL graft.

Matrix metalloproteinases (MMPs) play a central role in the degradation and remodeling of the extracellular matrix during healing and graft remodeling. Demirag and colleagues [41] performed bilateral ACL reconstruction with semitendinosus grafts in rabbits. Postoperatively, one knee joint was injected with α2-macroglobulin, which is an antagonist of synovial MMPs. The contralateral limb served as a control. On histologic analysis, the interface tissue in the treated group was more mature and contained numerous perpendicular collagen bundles (Sharpey's fibers). The ultimate load-to-failure was significantly greater in the treated group at 2 and 5 weeks. This study demonstrates that MMP inhibition can improve tendon graft healing in a bone tunnel.

BONE-TO-BONE HEALING IN ANTERIOR CRUCIATE LIGAMENT RECONSTRUCTION

When a bone-tendon-bone graft such as the patellar tendon is used for ACL reconstruction, graft fixation depends primarily on bone-to-bone healing. Bone-to-bone healing is widely accepted as the strongest form of healing in ACL reconstruction surgery. Studies have shown that the bone block of the graft first undergoes osteonecrosis, followed by rapid incorporation of surrounding host bone into the graft. Tomita and colleagues [5] compared healing of a soft tissue graft and of bone-patellar tendon-bone graft in a canine model. They confirmed that at 3 weeks the pull-out strength of the bone-patellar tendon-bone graft was significantly greater than that of the tendon graft, but at 6 weeks there was no significant difference. On histologic analysis of the bone-patellar tendon-bone healing site, they found that the graft was anchored by newly formed bone at 3 weeks, but a number of empty lacunae in the bone plug indicated osteonecrosis of the graft. On biomechanical testing at 3 weeks, all specimens failed at the graft–tunnel wall interface. At 6 weeks, the weakest point became the junction of the graft bone plug and the native insertion of the patellar tendon.

Papageorgiou and colleagues [4] compared bone-to-bone healing with tendon-to-bone healing in a goat ACL reconstruction model. Central-third bone-patellar tendon grafts were used to reconstruct the ACL. The bone portion of the graft was placed in the femoral tunnel, and the tendinous portion was secured in the tibial tunnel, allowing comparisons to be made between the two healing processes. All failures of the femur-ACL graft-tibia complex on biomechanical testing at 3 weeks occurred with graft pullout from the tibial tunnel indicating inferior healing of the tendon-to-bone site as compared with the bone-to-bone site. At 6 weeks, however, two of the seven grafts had midsubstance failures, whereas the remainder continued to be pulled out of the tibial tunnel. Histologic examination of the femoral tunnels (with bone-to-bone healing) at 3 weeks revealed a necrotic bone block surrounded by a thick interface of granulation tissue and a small amount of fibrous tissue. By 6 weeks, there was complete incorporation of the patellar bone block into the cancellous bone of the femoral tunnel. Tendon-to-bone healing in the tibial tunnel occurred in the same manner as described in previous studies.

A common misconception is that bone-to-bone healing of a bone plug in a bone tunnel occurs in the same manner as autologous bone grafting elsewhere in the body. Instead, several factors unique to ACL reconstruction may impede graft healing. First, in the clinical setting, the length of the tendon portion of most bone-patellar tendon-bone grafts is greater than the intra-articular ACL length. Thus a fair amount of tendon in the bone tunnel is concentrated at the tunnel aperture site (the end of the tunnel closest to the joint). Thus, graft healing at this important aperture site usually requires tendon-to-bone healing rather than bone-to-bone healing.

The second factor that may compromise healing in an intra-articular bone tunnel is the presence of synovial fluid at the graft–tunnel interface. Synovial fluid contains MMPs and other degradative enzymes that may impede healing and account for tunnel widening. To evaluate the healing behavior of an intra-articular bone tunnel continuously exposed to a synovial environment, Berg and colleagues [42] made bone tunnels in rabbit knees across the femur and tibia and left them empty. They found that these bone tunnels first heal at the areas furthest away from the joint. Healing of the empty bone tunnels then progressed slowly toward the joint. At 12 weeks, healing was slower and incomplete in the aperture (articular) segment, suggesting that synovial fluid may interfere with bone healing.

INTRA-ARTICULAR GRAFT HEALING

The ligamentization of a biologic graft is a complex process and takes a long time (Fig. 6). Regardless of the graft used, all intra-articular segments of tendon undergo a similar process. After surgery, the graft goes through an initial phase of acellular and avascular necrosis [43]; however, the collagen scaffold of the graft remains intact and unaffected. This phase is followed by cellular

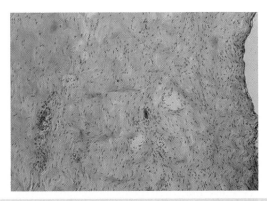

Fig. 6. Histology of intra-articular graft ligamentization in a rabbit ACL reconstruction. The graft has been repopulated by the host cells. (*Courtesy of* David Amiel, PhD, San Diego, California.)

repopulation by the host synovial cells [44]. After repopulation, revascularization occurs, followed by ligament maturation [45,46]. At the conclusion of this process, the graft is histologically and biochemically similar to the native ACL [46].

Panni and colleagues [47] nicely outlined the timing of the steps of intra-articular graft healing in rabbits that underwent ACL reconstructions with autologous patellar tendon grafts. At 2 weeks there were signs of necrosis and areas of fissuring of the fibrous tissue of the graft, although the collagen architecture remained intact. At 1 month, the intra-articular portion of the graft had undergone complete necrosis and was acellular, but again without significant alteration of the architecture of the collagen fibers. At 3 months, cellular repopulation with broad areas of vascular proliferation was seen. At 6 months, the number of cells in the graft had been reduced to a number more representative of normal ligament. At 9 months, the intra-articular portion of the graft had remodeled and was histologically similar to a normal ligament.

ALLOGRAFT HEALING IN ANTERIOR CRUCIATE LIGAMENT RECONSTRUCTION

Allografts are gaining popularity in ACL reconstruction. The allografts available for ACL reconstruction are bone-patellar tendon-bone, Achilles tendon, fascia lata, tibialis anterior and posterior tendons, and hamstring grafts. The main advantages of using allograft are the absence of donor-site morbidity and decreased operative time. Furthermore, multiple clinical studies have found no significant difference in the results of ACL reconstruction with patellar ligament autografts and allografts [48,49]. Although the strength of nonirradiated allografts is equal to that of autografts, graft incorporation and remodeling are slower for allografts and may make them more vulnerable to failure.

Several studies have examined the process by which an allograft heals after ACL reconstruction [43,50–52]. Allografts seem to heal in the same manner as their autograft counterparts but at a much slower rate. Allografts rely on tendon-to-bone healing and heal through the formation of fibrovascular scar tissue at the graft–tunnel interface with the eventual anchoring through the formation of Sharpey's fibers and new bone production [43,52]. Allografts that require bone-to-bone healing first undergo osteonecrosis of the bone plug portion of the graft, followed by incorporation of the graft by the surrounding cancellous bone from the tunnel [53].

The intra-articular portion of the allograft heals by acting as a collagen scaffold that subsequently is populated with host cells derived from the synovial fluid [43,54,55]. A study that used DNA probe analysis to evaluate donor cell survival in patellar ligament allografts used for ACL reconstruction in a goat model showed donor DNA was replaced entirely by host DNA within 4 weeks [56]. Graft revascularization then occurs predominately from the infrapatellar fat pad distally and from the posterior synovial tissues proximally [57]. Early revascularization begins 3 weeks after surgery with incomplete perfusion by 6 to 8 weeks in animal models [50]. Finally, collagen remodeling occurs in which the original large-diameter collagen fibrils are replaced with smaller-diameter fibrils [51]. As allografts undergo remodeling of the matrix, the tensile strength is reduced initially and then increases gradually until remodeling is complete [43,58,59]. Compared with autologous tissue, allografts lose more of their time-zero strength during remodeling; however, this difference has not been shown to be associated with poorer prognosis [51].

Several studies have shown that allografts heal at a slower rate than autografts. Jackson and colleagues [43] compared the healing of patellar tendon autografts with fresh allografts in a goat ACL reconstruction model. They found that although the structural and material properties of the autografts and allografts were similar at time zero, the allografts healed at a much slower rate. At 6 months, the autografts demonstrated better restraints to anterior-posterior displacement, twice the load-to-failure strength, a significant increase in cross-sectional area of the graft, and more small-diameter collagen fibrils than the allografts. The allografts demonstrated a greater decrease in their implantation structural properties, a slower rate of biologic incorporation, and the prolonged presence of an inflammatory response.

Because the relative hypocellularity of ligament allografts, the host immune response is limited. This immune response is elicited mostly by major histocompatibility class I and class II antigens that are present on donor cells within the ligament and bone components. The matrix of the allograft also may present antigenic epitotes that can incite an immune response. Freezing the allografts during graft preparation kills donor cells and may denature cell-surface histocompatibility antigens, resulting in decreased graft immunogenicity [45,60]. Studies, however, have shown that deep-frozen patellar ligament allografts used for ACL reconstruction can result in a detectable immune response because of the matrix antigens [61]. Rodrigo and colleagues [62] reported formation of antibodies against donor HLA antigens in the synovial fluid and serum of patients after ACL reconstruction using freeze-dried bone-patellar tendon-bone allografts. The clinical importance of such an immune response is unknown currently but may affect graft incorporation, revascularization, and graft remodeling.

References

[1] Hamner DL, Brown CH Jr, Steiner ME, et al. Hamstring tendon grafts for reconstruction of the anterior cruciate ligament: biomechanical evaluation of the use of multiple strands and tensioning techniques. J Bone Joint Surg Am 1999;81(4):549–57.

[2] Cooper DE, Deng XH, Burstein AL, et al. The strength of the central third patellar tendon graft. A biomechanical study. Am J Sports Med 1993;21(6):818–23, [discussion: 823–14].

[3] Kurosaka M, Yoshiya S, Andrish JT. A biomechanical comparison of different surgical techniques of graft fixation in anterior cruciate ligament reconstruction. Am J Sports Med 1987;15(3):225–9.

[4] Papageorgiou CD, Ma CB, Abramowitch SD, et al. A multidisciplinary study of the healing of an intraarticular anterior cruciate ligament graft in a goat model. Am J Sports Med 2001;29(5):620–6.

[5] Tomita F, Yasuda K, Mikami S, et al. Comparisons of intraosseous graft healing between the doubled flexor tendon graft and the bone-patellar tendon-bone graft in anterior cruciate ligament reconstruction. Arthroscopy 2001;17(5):461–76.

[6] Niyibizi C, Sagarrigo Visconti C, Gibson G, et al. Identification and immunolocalization of type X collagen at the ligament-bone interface. Biochem Biophys Res Commun 1996; 222(2):584–9.

[7] Sagarriga Visconti C, Kavalkovich K, Wu J, et al. Biochemical analysis of collagens at the ligament-bone interface reveals presence of cartilage-specific collagens. Arch Biochem Biophys 1996;328(1):135–42.

[8] Fujioka H, Thakur R, Wang GJ, et al. Comparison of surgically attached and non-attached repair of the rat Achilles tendon-bone interface. Cellular organization and type X collagen expression. Connect Tissue Res 1998;37(3–4):205–18.

[9] Goradia VK, Rochat MC, Grana WA, et al. Tendon-to-bone healing of a semitendinosus tendon autograft used for ACL reconstruction in a sheep model. Am J Knee Surg 2000;13(3): 143–51.

[10] Grana WA, Egle DM, Mahnken R, et al. An analysis of autograft fixation after anterior cruciate ligament reconstruction in a rabbit model. Am J Sports Med 1994;22(3):344–51.

[11] Rodeo SA, Arnoczky SP, Torzilli PA, et al. Tendon-healing in a bone tunnel. A biomechanical and histological study in the dog. J Bone Joint Surg Am 1993;75(12):1795–803.

[12] Kanazawa T, Soejima T, Murakami H, et al. An immunohistological study of the integration at the bone-tendon interface after reconstruction of the anterior cruciate ligament in rabbits. J Bone Joint Surg Br 2006;88(5):682–7.

[13] Sandberg MM, Aro HT, Vuorio EI. Gene expression during bone repair. Clin Orthop Relat Res 1993;289:292–312.

[14] Yamazaki S, Yasuda K, Tomita F, et al. The effect of intraosseous graft length on tendon-bone healing in anterior cruciate ligament reconstruction using flexor tendon. Knee Surg Sports Traumatol Arthrosc 2006;14(11):1086–93.

[15] Greis PE, Burks RT, Bachus K, et al. The influence of tendon length and fit on the strength of a tendon-bone tunnel complex. A biomechanical and histologic study in the dog. Am J Sports Med 2001;29(4):493–7.

[16] Singhatat W, Lawhorn KW, Howell SM, et al. How four weeks of implantation affect the strength and stiffness of a tendon graft in a bone tunnel: a study of two fixation devices in an extraarticular model in ovine. Am J Sports Med 2002;30(4):506–13.

[17] Kawamura S, Ying L, Kim HJ, et al. Macrophages accumulate in the early phase of tendon-bone healing. J Orthop Res 2005;23(6):1425–32.

[18] Hays P, Kawamura S, Deng X, et-al. The role of macrophages in early healing of a tendon graft in a bone tunnel: an experimental study in a rat anterior cruciate ligament reconstruction model. Presented at the Annual Meeting of the American Academy of Orthopaedic Surgeons. Chicago IL, March 22–26, 2006.

[19] Krivic A, Anic T, Seiwerth S, et al. Achilles detachment in rat and stable gastric pentadeca-peptide BPC 157: promoted tendon-to-bone healing and opposed corticosteroid aggravation. J Orthop Res 2006;24(5):982–9.

[20] Cohen DB, Kawamura S, Ehteshami JR, et al. Indomethacin and celecoxib impair rotator cuff tendon-to-bone healing. Am J Sports Med 2006;34(3):362–9.

[21] O'Keefe RJ, Tiyapatanaputi P, Xie C, et al. COX-2 has a critical role during incorporation of structural bone allografts. Ann N Y Acad Sci 2006;1068:532–42.

[22] Anderson K, Seneviratne AM, Izawa K, et al. Augmentation of tendon healing in an intra-articular bone tunnel with use of a bone growth factor. Am J Sports Med 2001;29(6): 689–98.

[23] Rodeo SA, Suzuki K, Deng XH, et al. Use of recombinant human bone morphogenetic protein-2 to enhance tendon healing in a bone tunnel. Am J Sports Med 1999;27(4): 476–88.

[24] Ma C, Kawamura S, Deng X, et al. Bone morphogenetic protein-signaling plays a role in tendon-to-bone healing: a study of rhBMP-2 and noggin. Am J Sports Med 2002;35(4): 597–604.

[25] Martinek V, Latterman C, Usas A, et al. Enhancement of tendon-bone integration of anterior cruciate ligament grafts with bone morphogenetic protein-2 gene transfer: a histological and biomechanical study. J Bone Joint Surg Am 2002;84-A(7):1123–31.

[26] Mihelic R, Pecina M, Jelic M, et al. Bone morphogenetic protein-7 (osteogenic protein-1) promotes tendon graft integration in anterior cruciate ligament reconstruction in sheep. Am J Sports Med 2004;32(7):1619–25.

[27] Tien YC, Chih TT, Lin JH, et al. Augmentation of tendon-bone healing by the use of calcium-phosphate cement. J Bone Joint Surg Br 2004;86(7):1072–6.

[28] Mutsuzaki H, Sakane M, Nakajima H, et al. Calcium-phosphate-hybridized tendon directly promotes regeneration of tendon-bone insertion. J Biomed Mater Res A 2004;70(2): 319–27.

[29] Dynybil C, Kawamura S, Kim HJ, et al. [The effect of osteoprotegerin on tendon-bone healing after reconstruction of the anterior cruciate ligament: a histomorphological and radiographical study in the rabbit]. Z Orthop Ihre Grenzgeb 2006;144(2): 179–86.

[30] Hantes ME, Mastrokalos DS, Yu J, et al. The effect of early motion on tibial tunnel widening after anterior cruciate ligament replacement using hamstring tendon grafts. Arthroscopy 2004;20(6):572–80.

[31] Rodeo SA, Kawamura S, Kim HJ, et al. Tendon healing in a bone tunnel differs at the tunnel entrance versus the tunnel exit: an effect of graft-tunnel motion? Am J Sports Med 2006;34(11):1790–800.

[32] Ouyang HW, Goh JC, Lee EH. Use of bone marrow stromal cells for tendon graft-to-bone healing: histological and immunohistochemical studies in a rabbit model. Am J Sports Med 2004;32(2):321–7.

[33] Lim JK, Hui J, Li L, et al. Enhancement of tendon graft osteointegration using mesenchymal stem cells in a rabbit model of anterior cruciate ligament reconstruction. Arthroscopy 2004;20(9):899–910.

[34] Yamazaki S, Yasuda K, Tomita F, et al. The effect of transforming growth factor-beta1 on intraosseous healing of flexor tendon autograft replacement of anterior cruciate ligament in dogs. Arthroscopy 2005;21(9):1034–41.

[35] Hildebrand KA, Woo SL, Smith DW, et al. The effects of platelet-derived growth factor-BB on healing of the rabbit medial collateral ligament. An in vivo study. Am J Sports Med 1998;26(4):549–54.

[36] Marui T, Niyibizi C, Georgescu HI, et al. Effect of growth factors on matrix synthesis by ligament fibroblasts. J Orthop Res 1997;15(1):18–23.

[37] Nagumo A, Yasuda K, Numazaki H, et al. Effects of separate application of three growth factors (TGF-beta1, EGF, and PDGF-BB) on mechanical properties of the in situ frozen-thawed anterior cruciate ligament. Clin Biomech 2005;20(3):283–90.

[38] Uggen JC, Dines J, Uggen CW, et al. Tendon gene therapy modulates the local repair environment in the shoulder. J Am Osteopath Assoc 2005;105(1):20–1.

[39] Weiler A, Forster C, Hunt P, et al. The influence of locally applied platelet-derived growth factor-BB on free tendon graft remodeling after anterior cruciate ligament reconstruction. Am J Sports Med 2004;32(4):881–91.

[40] Yoshikawa T, Tohyama H, Katsura T, et al. Effects of local administration of vascular endothelial growth factor on mechanical characteristics of the semitendinosus tendon graft after anterior cruciate ligament reconstruction in sheep. Am J Sports Med 2006;34(12):1918–25.

[41] Demirag B, Sarisozen B, Durak K, et al. The effect of alpha-2 macroglobulin on the healing of ruptured anterior cruciate ligament in rabbits. Connect Tissue Res 2004;45(1):23–7.

[42] Berg EE, Pollard ME, Kang Q. Interarticular bone tunnel healing. Arthroscopy 2001;17(2): 189–95.

[43] Jackson DW, Grood ES, Goldstein JD, et al. A comparison of patellar tendon autograft and allograft used for anterior cruciate ligament reconstruction in the goat model. Am J Sports Med 1993;21(2):176–85.

[44] Kleiner JB, Amiel D, Roux RD, et al. Origin of replacement cells for the anterior cruciate ligament autograft. J Orthop Res 1986;4(4):466–74.

[45] Arnoczky SP. Biology of ACL reconstructions: what happens to the graft? Instr Course Lect 1996;45:229–33.

[46] Arnoczky SP, Tarvin GB, Marshall JL. Anterior cruciate ligament replacement using patellar tendon. An evaluation of graft revascularization in the dog. J Bone Joint Surg Am 1982;64(2):217–24.

[47] Panni AS, Milano G, Lucania L, et al. Graft healing after anterior cruciate ligament reconstruction in rabbits. Clin Orthop Relat Res 1997;343:203–12.

[48] Bach BR Jr, Aadalen KJ, Dennis MG, et al. Primary anterior cruciate ligament reconstruction using fresh-frozen, nonirradiated patellar tendon allograft: minimum 2-year follow-up. Am J Sports Med 2005;33(2):284–92.

[49] Barrett G, Stokes D, White M. Anterior cruciate ligament reconstruction in patients older than 40 years: allograft versus autograft patellar tendon. Am J Sports Med 2005;33(10): 1505–12.

[50] Arnoczky SP, Warren RF, Ashlock MA. Replacement of the anterior cruciate ligament using a patellar tendon allograft. An experimental study. J Bone Joint Surg Am 1986;68(3): 376–85.

[51] Jackson DW, Corsetti J, Simon TM. Biologic incorporation of allograft anterior cruciate ligament replacements. Clin Orthop Relat Res 1996;324:126–33.

[52] Zhang CL, Fan HB, Xu H, et al. Histological comparison of fate of ligamentous insertion after reconstruction of anterior cruciate ligament: autograft vs allograft. Chin J Traumatol 2006;9(2):72–6.

[53] Harris NL, Indelicato PA, Bloomberg MS, et al. Radiographic and histologic analysis of the tibial tunnel after allograft anterior cruciate ligament reconstruction in goats. Am J Sports Med 2002;30(3):368–73.

[54] Jackson DW, Simon T. Assessment of donor cell survival in fresh allografts (ligament, tendon, and meniscus) using DNA probe analysis in a goat model. Iowa Orthop J 1993;13: 107–14.

[55] Min BH, Han MS, Woo JI, et al. The origin of cells that repopulate patellar tendons used for reconstructing anterior cruciate ligaments in man. J Bone Joint Surg Br 2003;85(5):753–7.
[56] Jackson DW, Simon TM, Kurzweil PR, et al. Survival of cells after intra-articular transplantation of fresh allografts of the patellar and anterior cruciate ligaments. DNA-probe analysis in a goat model. J Bone Joint Surg Am 1992;74(1):112–8.
[57] Nikolaou PK, Seaber AV, Glisson RR, et al. Anterior cruciate ligament allograft transplantation. Long-term function, histology, revascularization, and operative technique. Am J Sports Med 1986;14(5):348–60.
[58] Jackson DW, Grood ES, Arnoczky SP, et al. Freeze dried anterior cruciate ligament allografts. Preliminary studies in a goat model. Am J Sports Med 1987;15(4):295–303.
[59] Jackson DW, Grood ES, Cohn BT, et al. The effects of in situ freezing on the anterior cruciate ligament. An experimental study in goats. J Bone Joint Surg Am 1991;73(2):201–13.
[60] Noyes FR, Barber-Westin SD, Butler DL, et al. The role of allografts in repair and reconstruction of knee joint ligaments and menisci. Instr Course Lect 1998;47:379–96.
[61] Xiao Y, Parry DA, Li H, et al. Expression of extracellular matrix macromolecules around demineralized freeze-dried bone allografts. J Periodontol 1996;67(11):1233–44.
[62] Rodrigo J, Jackson D, Simon T, et al. The immune response to freeze-dried bone-tendon-bone ACL allografts in humans. Am J Knee Surg 1993;6:47–53.

Bone-Patella Tendon-Bone Autograft Anterior Cruciate Ligament Reconstruction

Robert J. Schoderbek, Jr, MD, Gehron P. Treme, MD,
Mark D. Miller, MD*

Department of Orthopaedic Surgery, University of Virginia Health Systems,
400 Ray C. Hunt Drive, Third Floor, Charlottesville, VA 22903, USA

The anterior cruciate ligament (ACL) serves an important stabilizing and biomechanical function for the knee. Reconstruction of the ACL remains one of the most commonly performed procedures in the field of sports medicine. Restoration of normal knee function and protection from further intra-articular injury, particularly injuries resulting from abnormal pivoting, drive continued research and development of new techniques for reconstruction. In preparation for ACL surgery, a patient must define and prioritize his/her functional expectations and desires for ACL reconstruction. Reconstruction of the ACL with bone-patella tendon-bone (BPTB) autograft secured with interference screw fixation has been the historical reference standard and remains the benchmark against which other methods are gauged.

An ideal ACL reconstruction technique would involve the use of a graft that is easily harvested, results in little harvest-site morbidity, has biomechanical properties equal or superior to those of the native ligament, possesses high initial strength and stiffness, can be secured predictably with rapid incorporation, and allows early aggressive rehabilitation while recreating the anatomy and function of the native knee [1–3]. Each of these topics has been the focus of endless research efforts during the past decade. Substantial advances have been made on all fronts, and current ACL reconstruction procedures address all these issues to some degree. The patients' expectations of returning to all activities at a performance level equal to preinjury levels have prompted evolution in graft selection and arthroscopic techniques. This evolution has occurred through improvements in arthroscopic skills and technology, advances in the understanding of the biomechanics of the knee, and development of sophisticated rehabilitation programs [1,4,5].

*Corresponding author. E-mail address: mdm3p@virginia.edu (M.D. Miller).

0278-5919/07/$ – see front matter
doi:10.1016/j.csm.2007.06.006

Reconstruction of the ACL with BPTB autograft secured with interference screws historically has been considered the reference standard for primary ACL reconstruction, and results of any other reconstructive technique are gauged against this method. Reconstruction of the ACL with BPTB autograft was first described by Jones in 1963 [1,2] and later was popularized by Clancy in 1982 [1,3]. Advantages of BPTB reconstruction include the superior biomechanical strength and stiffness of the graft, the ability to secure the graft firmly, the availability of bone-on-bone healing within both tunnels, and the ability to begin early, aggressive rehabilitation. Arthroscopically assisted one-incision ACL reconstruction has become the surgical technique of choice because of its shorter operating time, reduced postoperative morbidity, improved cosmesis, and quicker rehabilitation resulting from improved postoperative dynamic muscle function. Disadvantages of BPTB autograft ACL reconstruction are well documented and focus predominantly on graft-site morbidity. Disruption of the extensor mechanism, patella fracture, and patella baja and the increased risk of patellofemoral pain [6–8] have led surgeons to seek other graft options and have resulted in the development of newer fixation techniques. Other options include autograft hamstring and quadriceps tendon, as well as multiple types of allograft tissue.

This article reviews the reconstruction of the ACL with BPTB autograft including the surgical technique, rationale for BTPB use, and outcomes.

STAGES OF ANTERIOR CRUCIATE LIGAMENT RECONSTRUCTION

Preoperative Evaluation

Assessment of the knee joint before surgical intervention is critical to perform a successful procedure and is vital for a good result. Poor outcomes are associated with poor range of motion, weak quadriceps function, and excessive swelling. Before surgical intervention it is important to obtain a history of previous surgery or trauma to determine the best reconstructive technique for each specific patient.

After the decision has been made to proceed with surgery, care should be taken to optimize the patient's condition to provide the best chance for a good functional outcome. Surgery should be delayed until full range of motion (especially full extension), minimal swelling, optimal skin and soft tissue conditions, and good quadriceps activation have been demonstrated. Collateral ligament and meniscal injuries must be identified before reconstruction, because they may dictate earlier surgery with more involved operative intervention.

Appropriate preoperative radiographic assessment of the patellar tendon with a true lateral radiograph is important before surgical intervention to assure adequate graft length [1,9]. This assessment will help to avoid graft–tunnel mismatch and will allow the surgeon to choose an alternative graft choice if necessary.

It is important before graft harvest to note that ossicles can occur proximally or distally within the patella tendon, associated with Sinding-Larsen-Johansson or Osgood-Schlatter syndromes, respectively [10]. An ossicle in the harvested graft may compromise the tendon if removed or may shorten the relative length of the tendon to an unacceptable amount if not removed.

Examination Under Anesthesia

Reconstruction of the ACL can be performed under regional (spinal or epidural) or general anesthesia and can be supplemented with a femoral and/or sciatic nerve block to enhance postoperative analgesia [1,11]. After appropriate regional and/or general anesthesia has been instituted, and appropriate preoperative antibiotics have been delivered, a thorough examination under anesthesia with a complete knee examination is performed. The Lachman, anterior drawer, and pivot shift examinations are performed and graded for evaluation of the ACL. Posterior cruciate ligament (PCL) function is assessed with the posterior drawer. Varus and valgus stress with the knee in extension and 30° of flexion is checked for testing the lateral collateral ligament and medial collateral ligament, respectively. External rotation stability evaluating the continuity of the posterolateral corner and PCL is performed at 30° and 90°, respectively.

Patient Positioning

A nonsterile tourniquet is placed high on the thigh, and the operative leg is placed in a well-padded leg holder. The contralateral leg is placed in the lithotomy position in a well-leg holder that is padded with particular attention toward protection of the common peroneal nerve. The foot of the bed then is dropped, allowing the injured extremity to hang free with the knee in 90° of flexion and allowing flexion to 120° during the procedure (Fig. 1). Care should be taken to avoid excessive hip extension, which places the femoral nerve on stretch and can result in neurapraxia in longer surgeries. The operative leg then is prepped and draped using standard sterile technique. The leg is exsanguinated with a rubber bandage. The tourniquet is inflated to 300 mm Hg and remains inflated until the postoperative dressing is in place.

Diagnostic Arthroscopy

A diagnostic arthroscopy should be performed first if any findings on MRI, physical examination, or examination under anesthesia indicate a need for evaluation of the ACL to verify injury to the ligament. The standard anterolateral and anteromedial portals are made, and the suprapatellar pouch is entered. A limited fat pad débridement is performed to enhance visualization. The suprapatellar pouch and the medial and lateral gutters are examined for any evidence of injury or loose bodies. The medial and lateral compartments and the patellofemoral joint are evaluated to identify any articular cartilage damage or meniscus pathology. To help minimize operative time, injured menisci or damaged articular cartilage is addressed with repair or débridement as indicated while the graft preparation is being performed. Attention then is turned

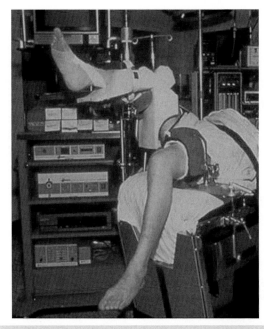

Fig. 1. Patient is positioned with the operative leg placed in a well-padded leg holder and the contralateral leg is placed in a well-leg holder. The foot of the bed is dropped allowing the injured extremity to hang free with the knee in 90° of flexion.

to the intercondylar notch. The PCL is examined and probed to check for tension. Verification of the ACL tear is made at this time. Full characterization of the tear is performed with the injured tissue photographed for the patient's record. Ligament laxity and an empty lateral wall should be assessed with a probe, and an anterior drawer test can be performed under direct visualization to assess ligament compromise.

Graft Harvest

Once an injury to the ACL has been confirmed by the diagnostic arthroscopy, or examination under anesthesia indicates an unequivocal ACL disruption, the patellar tendon autograft is harvested. The graft is harvested through a 4- to 6-cm incision that extends from the inferior pole of the patella to the tibial tubercle (Fig. 2). The incision should be placed just medial to midline to avoid the scar being directly over the prominent parts of the patella and tibial tubercle. Full-thickness skin and subcutaneous flaps are raised down through the retinacular layers to the paratenon. The paratenon is divided carefully and dissected off the tendon both medially and laterally, with care taken to preserve it so that it can be reapproximated later because of its importance in tendon defect regeneration and repair [1,12,13].

The patellar tendon width is measured, and an appropriate graft width is chosen. Although the majority of patellar tendons yield 10-mm grafts, 9-mm

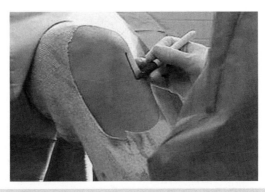

Fig. 2. The graft is harvested through a 4- to 6-cm incision that extends from the inferior pole of the patella to the tibial tubercle.

grafts should be harvested from tendons measuring less than 30 mm in width, and 11-mm grafts should be harvested from tendons wider than 38 mm [1]. The middle 10 cm of the tendon is identified, and a double-blade ACL patella tendon–harvesting knife or a single #10 surgical knife can be used for graft harvest. The graft should be harvested with the knee in flexion to keep the tendon under tension, to avoid cutting across the longitudinal oriented fibers of the patella tendon. Because the patella tendon is slightly externally rotated, the knife blade should be kept perpendicular to the tendon to avoid a skewed cutting of the tendon.

The tibial tubercle and patella bone blocks then should be measured and outlined for 20 to 25 mm in length and 10 mm in width with a single #10 surgical blade. A bone block is harvested with an oscillating saw in a rectangular fashion from the tibial tubercle cutting through the cortex to a depth of approximately 10 mm. A curved 0.25-inch osteotome then is used to make sure that the corners of the bone block are free from the remaining tubercle. The osteotome then is placed in the horizontal distal aspect of the cut, inserted to the desired depth, and levered to release the bone block from the remaining tubercle. The bone block is placed back into the tibial tubercle harvest site for protection, and attention is turned to the patella bone block.

A patella graft–harvesting retractor (Arthrex, Naples, Florida) is placed under the skin, and the patella is levered distally for better exposure of the patella bone block harvest site. Using the previously outlined dimensions, the oscillating saw is angled in a convergent manner for the longitudinal cuts to create a trapezoidal or triangular bone block. Caution should be used to avoid driving the saw too deep into the patella; avoiding cuts of excessive depth helps decrease the risk a patella fracture or chondral damage. The same 0.25-inch osteotome should be used to free the corners and periphery of the bone block to ensure an adequately sized bone block and to minimize the chance of developing a stress riser. The osteotome is used to lever the bone block from the surround patella, with care taken not to lever too forcefully. Thorough preparation of the cuts with the saw and gentle levering of the bone block at the proximal horizontal limb decrease the chance of perioperative fracture. The patella tendon graft then is carefully dissected free from the remaining patella tendon and surrounding fat pad. The BPTB graft should be brought carefully to the back table for preparation.

The bone blocks are sculpted using a small rongeur and an ACL graft-shaper clamp so that they fit through the appropriately sized hole of a sizing block (most commonly a 10-mm sizing block). The tibial bone block should be rounded at the leading end to assist in graft passage into the femoral tunnel. Any excess bone from either of the bone blocks can be saved and used to fill the harvest defect sites. A single hole is drilled using a 2-mm drill bit 5 to 8 mm from the end of the tibial bone block in an anterior-to-posterior direction, and a #5 nonabsorbable suture is threaded through the hole. The tibial tubercle end of the BTPB graft typically is placed in the femoral tunnel. Two evenly spaced holes then are made in the patella bone block perpendicular to each other, and #5 nonabsorbable sutures are threaded through each hole. This configuration helps protect at least one of the sutures from being cut during tibial tunnel fixation with interference screws. The bone–tendon junction at each end of the BTPB graft is marked with a surgical pen, and measurements of the graft are made for tunnel angulation. The measurements should include the entire graft length, tibial tubercle and patella bone block lengths, and patella tendon length (Fig. 3). The graft then is placed in a moist lap and is stored in a safe place on the back table.

Arthroscopy and Notch Preparation

If not previously executed, a diagnostic arthroscopy is performed while the graft is being prepared on the back table. Any meniscal or articular cartilage issues should be addressed at this time, but any chondral repair procedures, including osteochondral transplantation or microfracture, should be performed after the ACL is reconstructed so that arthroscopic visualization is optimized.

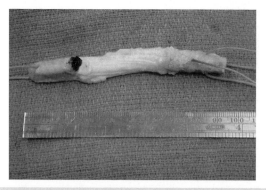

Fig. 3. Prepared patella tendon autograft with bone-tendon junction marked.

In addition, if an inside-out meniscus repair is performed, the sutures are tied following the graft fixation. The remnant ACL is excised using a shaver and biters to allow full access to the lateral wall of the intercondylar notch and to prevent impingement of the graft on soft tissue. The tibial footprint of the ACL insertion site is cleared, making sure to leave an outline for proper tibial tunnel placement. All soft tissue is cleared from the lateral wall and roof of the intercondylar notch lateral to the PCL attachment, with care taken to avoid damage to the PCL throughout the débridement. After the soft tissue has been débrided adequately, a large burr and rasp are used to complete the notchplasty.

Notchplasty

It is important to create a smooth tunnel-shaped notch that allows easy visualization and access to the posterior notch for accurate femoral tunnel placement and that avoids impingement of the ACL graft on the lateral wall and roof. Identification of the over-the-top position is important for appropriate femoral tunnel position (Fig. 4). Care should be taken to avoid mistaking anterior irregularities of the notch roof, also known as "resident's ridge," for the over-the-top position. This mistake will lead to an anteriorly placed femoral tunnel that can result in graft impingement and failure [14].

Many surgeons perform a conservative notchplasty (less than 5 mm of bone) to enhance visualization of critical anatomic landmarks and to decrease impingement of the graft on the roof and lateral wall of the notch while avoiding the pitfalls of overresection, which has been linked to patellofemoral dysfunction [15,16]. A small amount of bone is removed from the superior and lateral aspect of the notch, giving the notch an appearance of a tunnel. A fringe of white periosteal tissue, denoting the junction of the femur and the posterior joint capsule, usually can be seen posteriorly when the over-the-top position

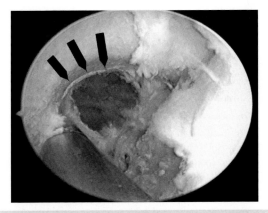

Fig. 4. Over-the-top position with a fringe of white periosteal tissue (*black arrows*) denoting the junction of the femur and the posterior joint capsule.

has been identified. An arthroscopic probe should be used to verify this position.

The amount of notch preparation needed for successful ACL reconstruction remains controversial. With debate persisting about the role of notch width in rupture of the native ACL, the need to widen the notch before graft placement remains unclear. On the other hand, the ACL graft must be placed in the correct location to maximize the benefit of the reconstruction, and identification of consistent surgical landmarks is critical to the success of the procedure. Most surgeons agree that at least enough bone and soft tissue should be resected from the notch to ensure proper graft position.

TUNNEL PLACEMENT

Proper placement and reaming of the tibial and femoral tunnels is paramount to achieve a graft that is isometric through a full range of motion and to control anterior translation and rotational stability of the knee. Recognition of pivot control as the main goal of ACL reconstruction and improved knowledge of the true anatomic insertion of the ACL on the femur has led to the placement of the femoral tunnel farther down the face of the intercondylar notch than previously described [3,17]. The tunnel should be located nearer the 10 o'clock position on the femur for the right knee (the 2 o'clock position for the left knee) for optimal results and to resist rotatory loads more effectively [3,13].

The placement of the femoral tunnel, however, is predicated largely on the position of the tibial tunnel when a transtibial technique is used. This fact has led to some changes in tibial tunnel location. A more medial tibial starting point changes the trajectory of the tunnel and allows placement of the femoral over-the-top guide farther down the notch face, creating the ideal ACL graft location and maximizing the benefits of reconstruction [17,18]. The starting point on the tibia should be midpoint from inferior to superior with respect to the tibial tubercle harvest site and midpoint between the tibial tubercle and the postero-medial edge of the tibia. Placing a tunnel too far medial may compromise the superficial and medial collateral ligament, and placing it too central creates a vertical tunnel. A vertically placed tunnel compromises the femoral tunnel placement and may lead to a graft that provides anterior restraint to translation but insufficiently controls rotation.

Tibial Tunnel Placement

A commercially available guide can be used to ensure proper entry of the tibial tunnel into the joint. Landmarks for placement of the tibial tunnel are well defined and include a position 7 mm anterior to the fibers of the PCL, the up-slope of the lateral face of the medial tibial intercondylar eminence, the posterior aspect of the anterior horn of the lateral meniscus, and the center of the native ACL footprint [1,19,20]. Careful attention to these landmarks is critical, because a tibial tunnel that is too far anterior or lateral results in intercondylar notch impingement; whereas a tunnel too far posterior leads to a vertical graft that allows anterior laxity and poor pivot control. In the sagittal plane the tunnel must be angled posteriorly so that the graft does not impinge on the intercondylar roof. A lateral radiograph of the knee in extension should show the entry of the tibial tunnel into the joint posterior to Blumensaat's line (the roof of the intercondylar notch). In the coronal plane, the tibial tunnel should be angled 70° to the medial tibial plateau to produce an appropriate angle for femoral tunnel drilling and to recreate the oblique nature of the native ACL [1,21].

The elbow or tip aimer of the ACL tibial guide is placed through the anteromedial portal, and the tip of the guide is placed at the landmarks previously mentioned (Fig. 5). The angle of the guide is usually set to 50° to 55°. The calculations of N + 2-mm and N + 7° (with N as the length the tendinous portion of the patella tendon graft) are used to help estimate the length of the tibial tunnel and angle of the guide required to fit the patella tendon graft, respectively [22–26]. These calculations can be used as guidelines to help avoid a graft–tunnel mismatch, but these guidelines are not infallible, and intraoperative adjustments based on surgical judgment are needed to maximize tunnel placement.

The guide pin is inserted, starting along the medial aspect of the anterior surface of the tibia between the tibial tubercle and the posteromedial edge of the tibia. After the guide pin is inserted into the proper location, the soft tissues on the tibia are reflected, and an appropriate-sized acorn reamer based on graft size (usually 10 mm) is used to ream the tunnel line to line. A curette should be placed over the top of the tip of the guide pin to protect the articular cartilage and PCL from injury. A cannulated bone-reaming collector or 10-mm graft sizer should be placed over top of the reamer to help collect excess bone to use as bone graft at the harvest sites. The reamer is advanced until resistance is felt or the guide pin starts to rotate, indicating that the subchondral bone of the tibial plateau has been reached. Then the inflow pump is turned off, and the

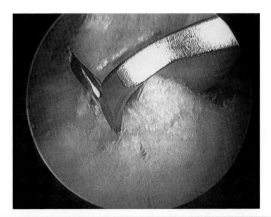

Fig. 5. The boom of the ACL tibial guide with guidewire placed 7 mm anterior to the fibers of the PCL, the upslope of the lateral face of the medial tibial intercondylar eminence, the posterior aspect of the anterior horn of the lateral meniscus, and the center of the native ACL footprint.

reamer is advanced further to penetrate into the joint. The reamer then should be removed, and all excess bone graft from drilling the tibial tunnel is collected to use as bone graft [27]. Finally, the arthroscopic shaver is used to débride all soft tissue surrounding the tibial tunnel to allow easier graft passage and to smooth the posterior edge of the tunnel to preventing graft abrasion.

Femoral Tunnel Placement

Placement of the femoral guide pin can be accomplished in a transtibial fashion or through the inferomedial arthroscopic portal (medial portal technique). Both techniques have advocates. Proponents of the portal method cite the ability to place the guide pin lower on the intercondylar notch as a major advantage. Surgeons preferring the transtibial technique argue that improved visualization and consistent placement using the femoral guide are distinct advantages. As mentioned previously, placement of the femoral pin low on the intercondylar notch is facilitated by starting the tibial tunnel on the medial aspect of the tibia. The authors prefer the transtibial technique for femoral tunnel placement.

The over-the-top position should be well defined, and a commercially available over-the-top offset guide places the guidewire at the desired position by using the predetermined offset (Fig. 6). This offset is calculated by adding the radius of the planned tunnel size to the 1 to 2 mm of desired posterior wall. The femoral offset guide is advanced through the tibial tunnel, and the tongue of the device is placed in the 10 o'clock over-the-top position to recreate better the original femoral footprint of the native ACL. A Beath needle (a long guidewire with an eyelet at one end) is inserted through the offset guide and is drilled through the anterolateral femur with the knee hyperflexed (Fig. 7) to ensure that the Beath needle exits through the distal thigh, especially when using the leg holder and there is less room for the needle to exit. It is imperative that the position of the knee not change until the Beath needle is removed with graft passage to ensure that it does not bend. Bending can result in shearing of the

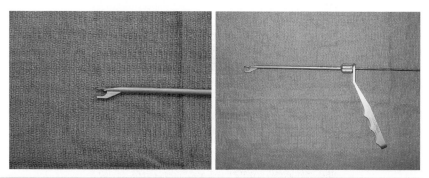

Fig. 6. A commercially available over-the-top offset guide (Smith and Nephew, Andover, Massachusetts) places the guidewire at the desired position by using the predetermined offset.

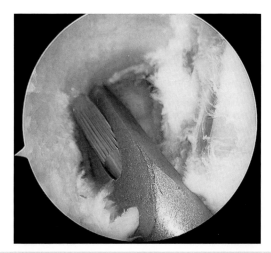

Fig. 7. The tongue of the femoral offset guide is placed in the over-the-top position, and the Beath needle is drilled through the anterolateral femur.

needle with reaming. Next, the offset guide is removed, and the guidewire should be assessed for correct placement and to ensure that there will be appropriate amount of posterior wall after reaming. A 10-cm acorn reamer is placed over the guidewire, and the femoral tunnel is drilled to a depth of 30 to 35 mm. The tunnel then should be reassessed for an intact posterior wall (Fig. 8). The shaver is used to clear all excess bone debris out of the tunnel and posterior notch.

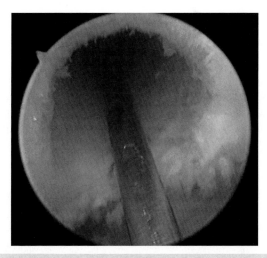

Fig. 8. Femoral tunnel with intact posterior wall.

Graft Passage

The BTPB graft should be obtained from the back table, and the sutures from the patella bone block (the bone block that will be secured in the tibial tunnel) should be clamped to the drape close to the knee to ensure that the graft will not fall to the ground. The single-suture limbs that are in the tibial bone block should be threaded through eyelet of the Beath needle, and the needle should be pulled out of the anterolateral thigh with the suture. The knee can be brought back to a neutral position, and the graft should be pulled carefully into the knee. With the help of a probe, the tibial tubercle bone block should be directed into the femoral tunnel with the cancellous portion facing anteriorly. If the fit of the bone block is very tight, it may need to be coerced into the tunnel with the probe or tapped gently with a large Association for Osteosynthesis (AO) screwdriver or rasp. If there are significant problems getting the bone block into the femoral tunnel, one should make sure that the patella bone block is not hindering the graft's advancement in the distal end of the tibial tunnel.

FIXATION

The primary advantage of BPTB graft has long been the ability to secure the graft with excellent initial strength and stiffness and the resultant bone-to-bone healing. Many methods of femoral fixation have been used over time, including extracortical suspensory systems, screw and washer constructs, and interference screws. Interference screw fixation has greater initial fixation strength than other fixation techniques and allows the desired bone-to-bone healing [1,28–30]. Both metal and bioabsorbable screws have been used and provide equivalent fixation strength [1,28,31–36]. The advantage of bioabsorbable interference screws is the apparent absorption of the material over time, facilitating revision surgery if necessary [36]. This concept of material absorption is controversial: studies using CT and MRI scans indicate that the material may not resorb completely and may be replaced by fibrous tissue [1,36,37]. This process does not seem to change the fixation strength of the bioabsorbable screws or the ability to allow bone-on-bone healing.

When deciding on screw diameter, the perceived quality of the bone and tightness of fit must be assessed. A 7-mm screw is used primarily in the femoral tunnel when it is believed that there is good-quality bone and a tight-fitting 10-mm bone block. A 9-mm screw should be used be when there is poorer-quality bone or a looser-fitting bone block. A 9-mm screw is used primarily in the tibial tunnel because of the softer metaphyseal bone fixation. It also is important to keep at least 10 mm of bone plug in contact with the interference screw to obtain maximum bone-holding potential and to minimize peak load to failure [38].

To reduce the chance of graft damage by the interference screw and poor graft fixation caused by screw divergence, the screw must be placed as parallel to the bone blocks as possible, ideally with a divergence of less than 30° between bone plug and screw [1,39–41].

Femoral Tunnel Fixation

For the femoral interference screw to be placed parallel to the bone block, the knee must be hyperflexed. If it is difficult to obtain parallel placement of the interference screw through the anteromedial portal, the portal can be enlarged distally, or the screw can be placed through the patella tendon defect. A tunnel notcher (Arthrex, Naples, Florida) is used to create an antirotation slot at the anterior interface between the femoral bone block and tunnel to assist with placement of the guidewire and interference screw.

It is important to place the guidewire in the antirotation slot and to advance it into the femoral tunnel. With the knee hyperflexed and with equal tension placed on the both ends of the graft through the sutures (making sure that the graft does not advance with screw placement), the interference screw is inserted until its end is flush with the end of the bone block (Fig. 9). Failure to advance the screw to past the bone–soft tissue interface may result in graft abrasion by the screw. Tension should be placed on the tibial bone block sutures to check the strength of the femoral fixation. No slippage of the graft or motion of the screw should be observed, indicating adequate fixation.

Arthroscopic assessment for graft impingement on the lateral wall or intercondylar roof should be performed with the graft under tension and the knee brought through a full range of motion, in particular full extension (Fig. 10). Any evidence of impingement should be addressed carefully at this time. The knee should be cycled though a full range of motion 15 to 20 times to remove any crimps from the graft complex before tibial fixation. Abnormal graft pistoning also should be assessed while cycling the knee and by feeling for pistoning of graft at the tibial tunnel opening. A graft that pistons more than 2 mm indicates poor tunnel placement and lack of isometry [1].

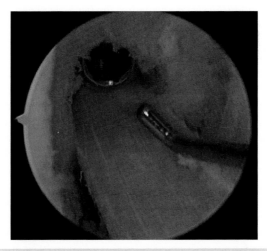

Fig. 9. ACL reconstruction with BPTB autograft with metallic screw flush with edge of bone block.

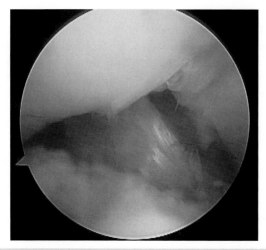

Fig. 10. With the knee in full extension, no graft impingement is noted with either the lateral wall or intercondylar roof.

Tibial Tunnel Fixation

Debate persists as to the proper position of the knee and tension on the graft at the time of tibial fixation. Recommendations vary as to the optimal amount of knee flexion when securing the graft. Studies have demonstrated that the ACL experiences maximum load at full extension and lowest load at 30° of flexion [42–44]. Overtensioning of the graft in flexion increases stability but also increases the risk of graft stretching as the knee reaches full extension. A graft placed under maximum tension in extension results in a stable reconstruction and decreases the likelihood of elongation during knee range of motion. After cycling the knee with the femoral fixation in place, the authors place the graft under maximal tension with the knee in full extension before securing it to the tibia. An appropriately sized interference screw then is placed over a guidewire anterior to the bone block. Greater tension on the graft can be obtained with the knee flexed to 20° to 30°, a posterior drawer applied to the proximal tibia, and maximal tension applied to the sutures. The knee then should be brought through a full range of motion to make sure that full extension can be obtained and tested for stability with the Lachman's and pivot shift tests to ensure a stable reconstruction. The graft should be probed to ensure appropriate tension. A second point of fixation with a staple or screw washer construct can be placed if fixation quality is a concern.

Any excess bone from the bone block sculpting or tibial tunnel excavation is packed in the patella and tibial tubercle harvest sites and tamped into place. The patella defect is closed with 0-Vicryl (Ethicon, Somerville, New Jersey) interrupted buried sutures. The paratenon is reapproximated over the extent of the incision to keep the bone graft in place and to help enhance healing and apparent regeneration of the patella tendon defect. The remainder of the incision is closed in layers with 0 and 2-0 Vicryl suture and a running Prolene (Ethicon, Somerville, New Jersey) for the skin. If present, the anteromedial and anterolateral portal sites are closed with 2-0 nylon suture. The tourniquet is released, a sterile dressing is applied, and an elastic bandage is placed from the toes past the knee. In the absence of meniscal repair, patients are allowed to bear weight without a brace, as tolerated, in the immediate postoperative period and are discharged home from the ambulatory care center.

Graft–Tunnel Mismatch

The surgeon needs to have alternate fixation techniques in his/her repertoire to deal with graft–tunnel mismatch when the bone block extrudes through the distal aspect of the tibial tunnel. Minimal extrusion can be treated by recessing the femoral bone block by 5 mm further into the femoral canal, taking care not to recess more than 5 mm because doing so can compromise of the tendinous portion of the graft and make placement of the interference screw difficult. Twisting the graft also can help to shorten its length. A study by Auge [45] showed that at 630° of external rotation, approximately 25% shortening of the collagenous portion of the graft can be achieved. Significant graft extrusion with most of the bone block extruding from the tibial tunnel can be treated by creating a trough at the mouth of the tibial tunnel. The graft then can be held in place with a staple, and the sutures can be tied over a post to obtain a second point of fixation. Barber [46] described a technique of "flipping" of the bone block 180° onto the tendon, which shortens the graft by the length of the bone block, and fixing it within the tibial tunnel with a bioabsorbable screw.

REHABILITATION

The first and most important step in rehabilitation of an ACL reconstruction is avoiding preoperative stiffness. Patients should be evaluated for range of motion at the time of the initial visit with particular attention paid to the ability to achieve full extension. Any concern by the physician regarding the patient's preoperative motion should be addressed by a referral to a physical therapist for aggressive therapy for knee range of motion and a repeat clinical evaluation before the surgery. The patient should be informed that surgery will be postponed until these motion goals are met. Insisting on adequate preoperative range of motion increases the likelihood that the patient will achieve acceptable postoperative motion and invests the patient from the beginning in the treatment needed to achieve a successful outcome.

After surgery, a supervised rehabilitation protocol is instituted immediately. To enhance compliance, both the patient and therapist receive a copy of the protocol. In the absence of meniscal repair, patients are allowed to bear weight as tolerated without a brace. If meniscal repair is performed, the patient is placed in a hinged knee brace with a range of motion of zero to 90° of flexion and kept in partial weight bearing for 6 weeks after surgery. Proprioceptive training and closed-chain exercises are started immediately with proper quadriceps recruitment an early goal. Treadmill walking, stationary bicycle, and aquatic therapy are stressed to increase knee motion, strengthen the extremity, and begin gait training as part of the initial regimen. At 5 to 6 weeks after surgery conventional weight machines are used, and the patient begins to use an elliptical trainer. Plyometric exercise is started 8 weeks after surgery and is continued until the end of rehabilitation. Patients may start jogging 12 weeks postoperatively and return to sports-specific training as progression with the therapist indicates over the next 4 weeks. Return to sport is allowed when the following criteria are met: quadriceps difference of less than 15% on isokinetic testing, power difference less than 15%, peak torque-to-body weight ratio greater than 80%, hamstring-to-quadriceps ratio greater than 60%, 85% or better on scores of functional tests, no pain, no swelling, ability to perform desired activity at full speed, and, finally, physician agreement.

COMPLICATIONS

Despite the biomechanical strength and stiffness that this graft provides for ACL reconstruction, it can have complications. Most of the attention has focused on graft harvest morbidity. Kneeling pain is the one complaint that is unique to patella tendon reconstruction and frequently persists [1,26,47–52]. It is important that the patients be informed of this possibility before surgical intervention. Patellofemoral pain (anterior knee pain) continues to be an issue, although rehabilitation techniques have improved [1,26,47–52]. Rates of reported patellofemoral pain after BTPB ACL autograft reconstruction range from 3% to 50% [1,51,53–55], but patellofemoral pain also has been reported in 22% of ACL-deficient knees and in 20% of hamstring reconstructions [1,56]. Shelbourne and Trumper [57] found no difference in the incidence of patellofemoral pain in 602 BPTB autograft ACL reconstructions and 122 control knees with no surgical intervention. They concluded that patellofemoral pain is not inherent to BPTB harvest and that the incidence of pain can be minimized with emphasis on restoration of hyperextension. Disturbance of anterior knee sensitivity caused by intraoperative injury to the infrapatellar branch of the saphenous nerve is a known complication associated with graft harvest. Patella tendonitis is present in 10% of patients in the first 3 to 6 months of rehabilitation but usually resolves after the first year [1,58,59]. Patella tendon shortening of more than 3 mm has been observed in more than 30% of patients. This finding may influence the patellofemoral joint by altering the alignment and pressure distribution [60–62]. Reconstruction failure, defined as pathologic laxity of the reconstructed ACL, has been reported to range between 10% and 29%. This complication most commonly results from an anteriorly placed tibial tunnel causing the graft to impinge on the roof of the intercondylar notch during full knee extension [4,14,63–65]. Extensor mechanism disruption, specifically patella tendon rupture, is a rare but reported complication that typically occurs early in the postoperative period [66]. Patella fractures, reported to have an incidence of 1.3%, are less likely with careful technique and have been shown to cause minimal residual sequelae when managed appropriately [1,67]. Patella fracture is thought to occur from the redistribution of the surface strain after bone is removed from the inferior aspect of the patella, resulting in a greater strain adjacent to the upper border of the bone block. Loss of full motion and knee extensor strength deficits have been reported to occur at 60° to 95° and to improve with continued rehabilitation [68,69]. Radiographic osteoarthritic changes are related to the status of the meniscus at the time of surgery and can be diminished if reconstruction is performed before chronic meniscal changes occur [1,70,71].

OUTCOMES

Rupture of the ACL leads to abnormal knee kinematics and predisposes the joint to degenerative changes. Activities that demand cutting, pivoting, and quick changes in direction can be difficult and lead to instability with a knee that is ACL deficient. Arthroscopically assisted ACL reconstruction facilitates early recovery and rehabilitation, allows an early return to preinjury activity, improves patient discomfort, and diminishes the chances of osteoarthritic changes in the knee. The ideal graft should reproduce the complex anatomy and biomechanical properties of the native ACL, permit strong and secure fixation to allow early rehabilitation, promote rapid biologic incorporation, and minimize donor-site morbidity. The appropriate graft for ACL reconstruction depends on numerous factors, including tissue availability, the patient's activity level and desires, and the surgeon's experience and philosophy [2].

Arthroscopic ACL reconstruction with BPTB autograft historically has been seen as the reference standard for restoring functional knee stability, with successful results in 85% to 95% of cases [3,4,72]. The advantages of BPTB reconstruction include the superior biomechanical strength and stiffness of the graft, the ability to secure the graft firmly with the availability of bone-to-bone healing within both tunnels, and the ability to begin early, aggressive rehabilitation [1,3,71].

Improvements in surgical techniques, fixation devices, and tensioning techniques and diminished complications associated with harvest-site morbidity have increased the use of hamstring autograft for ACL reconstruction. Initial reports of hamstring autograft stated that they lacked the strength or stiffness of native and BTPB autograft ACLs, leading to early graft failure. The use of a quadrupled hamstring graft and improvements in fixation and strength have increased the use of this graft source for ACL reconstruction. Many prospective, randomized, controlled studies during the past 2 decades have compared BPTB autografts and hamstring autografts. The majority of the studies have shown no statistically significant differences between the autograft techniques in Tegner activity level, Lysholm score, knee laxity measurements with physical examination and KT-1000 recordings, functional outcome, and International Knee Documentation Committee (IKDC) classification [21,47,58,59,73–75]. The only statistically significant finding in the majority of the studies was greater patellofemoral pain associated with BPTB autograft because of graft-site harvest [26,47–49,58,59,75,76]. A few of the studies showed flexion deficits with hamstring autograft and extension deficits with BTPB autograft [21,47,48,74].

The biomechanical properties of the BPTB autograft have been studied and compared with the native ACL and other ACL graft choices [2,48,77–79]. Noyes and colleagues [77] studied the mechanical and structural properties of the native ACL and different tendons that could be used for reconstruction. They reported the mean ultimate tensile strength (failure load) and stiffness of the native ACL to be 1725 newtons (N) and 182 N/mm respectively [77]. The BPTB autograft, with average width of 14 mm, was found to have a mean ultimate tensile strength and stiffness of 2900 N and 685 N/mm, 168% of the strength and four times the stiffness of the native ACL [2,48,77]. Cooper and colleagues [79] reported the ultimate tensile strength of a 10-mm BPTB autograft to be 2977 N. The initial studies testing hamstring autografts for strength and stiffness showed the hamstring graft to be weaker than BPTB graft, but these studies used two-stranded hamstring autografts. A subsequent study by Hamner and colleagues [80], using equally tensioned quadrupled hamstring autograft, reported mean ultimate tensile strength and stiffness of 4090 N and 776 N/mm. This study showed that the tensile properties of qua-druple-stranded hamstring autografts are additive when the strands are tensioned equally and that equal tensioning is needed for the graft to achieve optimal biomechanical properties [2,48,52,80].

A few prospective randomized studies have reported increased laxity with hamstring autograft. Beynnon and colleagues [81] showed decreased flexion strength and increased knee laxity in patients treated with two-strand hamstring autograft compared with those treated with BPTB autograft. Anderson and colleagues [82], in a study with 2-year follow-up comparing BPTB autograft, a semitendinosus and gracilis with iliotibial band extra-articular procedure, and semitendinosus and gracilis autograft alone reported increased knee laxity in both hamstring groups and higher IKDC ratings with the BPTB autograft. A recent study by Feller and colleagues [76] showed 88% of the BPTB group versus 68% of the hamstring tendon group returning to level I or II activities at the 3-year follow-up. Aglietti and colleagues [64] concluded that BPTB autograft was preferred because return of stability was more reliable.

Because of the numerous studies during the past 2 decades that have compared BPTB autograft with hamstring tendon autograft, a few meta-analyses have been completed on the subject in recent years. In 2001, Yunes and colleagues [26] performed a meta-analysis reviewing four studies with a total of 411 subjects and reported that the BPTB autograft group had significantly less laxity than the hamstring group as measured by the KT-1000 arthrometer and reported a 18% higher rate of "return to preinjury level of activity." In 2003 Freedman and colleagues [49] pooled data from 34 studies with a total of 1976 subjects (1348 BPTB and 628 hamstring) and showed increased patel-lofemoral pain, less laxity, lower rates of graft failure, improved static stability, and higher patient satisfaction in the BPTB autograft group. In 2005, Goldblatt and colleagues [48] collected data from 11 studies with a total of 1039 subjects (515 BPTB and 524 hamstring) and showed the previously mentioned complications of anterior knee pain, increased kneeling pain, flexion deficit with hamstring autograft, and extension deficit with BPTB autograft were present in patients who had undergone ACL reconstruction. The incidence of instability was reported as being not significantly different in the BPTB and hamstring autografts, but BPTB was more likely to result in reconstructions that had a normal Lachman examination, pivot shift examination, KT-1000 side-to-side difference of less than 3 mm, and fewer instances of significant flexion loss. Also in 2005, Prodromos and colleagues [52] collected data from 64 studies showing that the quadrupled hamstring ACL reconstruction produces higher stability rates than BPTB and is fixation dependent.

SUMMARY

Clearly, the controversy over the best graft choice for ACL reconstruction is not over. Additionally, despite the recent increase in the use of various soft tissue graft sources, BPTB autograft has not been displaced as the reconstruction graft option against which all others are measured. No choice of graft is ideal for all patients, and the modern surgeon should be skillful in using more than one type of graft to allow the surgeon and the patient the opportunity to make an educated decision about the most suitable graft. A patient must define and prioritize his/her functional expectations and desires for ACL reconstruction. A few generalized conclusions have been made during the past few decades from the multiple studies that have tried to determine the best graft for different groups of patients. Multiple studies showing statistically significant findings of patellofemoral pain associated with BPTB graft harvest indicate that patients who perform significant amounts of kneeling, occupationally or religiously, should consider a graft selection other than BPTP autograft for ACL reconstruction [2]. BPTB autograft is favored for patients who have high demands for overall stability, who need to return to level I or II sports, or who have a chronic ACL disruption [1–3,26,47,48]. BPTB ACL reconstruction results in reproducible and dependable return to function that has stood the test of time. Although other graft options exist, BPTB autograft remains an excellent option when used in the appropriate clinical context.

References

[1] Gladstone JN, Andrews JR. Endoscopic anterior cruciate ligament reconstruction with patella tendon autograft. Orthop Clin North Am 2002;33(4):701–15.
[2] Miller SL, Gladstone JN. Graft selection in anterior cruciate ligament reconstruction. Orthop Clin North Am 2002;33(4):675–83.
[3] Cain EL Jr, Clancy WG Jr. Anatomic endoscopic anterior cruciate ligament reconstruction with patella tendon autograft. Orthop Clin North Am 2002;33(4):717–25.
[4] Shelbourne KD, Klootwyk TE, Wilckens JH, et al. Ligament stability two to six years after anterior cruciate ligament reconstruction with autogenous patellar tendon graft and participation in accelerated rehabilitation program. Am J Sports Med 1995;23(5): 575–9.
[5] Shelbourne KD, Nitz P. Accelerated rehabilitation after anterior cruciate ligament reconstruction. Am J Sports Med 1990;18(3):292–9.

[6] Ejerhed L, Kartus J, Sernert N, et al. Patellar tendon or semitendinosus tendon autografts for anterior cruciate ligament reconstruction? A prospective randomized study with a two-year follow-up. Am J Sports Med 2003;31(1):19–25.

[7] Laxdal G, Kartus J, Hansson L, et al. A prospective randomized comparison of bone-patellar tendon-bone and hamstring grafts for anterior cruciate ligament reconstruction. Arthroscopy 2005;21(1):34–42.

[8] Laxdal G, Sernert N, Ejerhed L, et al. A prospective comparison of bone-patellar tendon-bone and hamstring tendon grafts for anterior cruciate ligament reconstruction in male patients. Knee Surg Sports Traumatol Arthrosc 2007;15(2):115–25.

[9] McAllister DR, Bergfeld JA, Parker RD, et al. A comparison of preoperative imaging techniques for predicting patellar tendon graft length before cruciate ligament reconstruction. Am J Sports Med 2001;29(4):461–5.

[10] McCarroll JR, Shelbourne KD, Patel DV. Anterior cruciate ligament reconstruction in athletes with an ossicle associated with Osgood-Schlatter's disease. Arthroscopy 1996;12(5): 556–60.

[11] Mulroy MF, Larkin KL, Batra MS, et al. Femoral nerve block with 0.25% or 0.5% bupivacaine improves postoperative analgesia following outpatient arthroscopic anterior cruciate ligament repair. Reg Anesth Pain Med 2001;26(1):24–9.

[12] Kohn D, Sander-Beuermann A. Donor-site morbidity after harvest of a bone-tendon-bone patellar tendon autograft. Knee Surg Sports Traumatol Arthrosc 1994;2(4):219–23.

[13] Sanchis-Alfonso V, Subias-Lopez A, Monteagudo-Castro C, et al. Healing of the patellar tendon donor defect created after central-third patellar tendon autograft harvest. A long-term histological evaluation in the lamb model. Knee Surg Sports Traumatol Arthrosc 1999; 7(6):340–8.

[14] Almekinders LC, Chiavetta JB, Clarke JP. Radiographic evaluation of anterior cruciate ligament graft failure with special reference to tibial tunnel placement. Arthroscopy 1998; 14(2):206–11.

[15] Asahina S, Muneta T, Ezura Y. Notchplasty in anterior cruciate ligament reconstruction: an experimental animal study. Arthroscopy 2000;16(2):165–72.

[16] Hame SL, Markolf KL, Hunter DM, et al. Effects of notchplasty and femoral tunnel position on excursion patterns of an anterior cruciate ligament graft. Arthroscopy 2003;19(4): 340–5.

[17] Loh JC, Fukuda Y, Tsuda E, et al. Knee stability and graft function following anterior cruciate ligament reconstruction: comparison between 11 o'clock and 10 o'clock femoral tunnel placement. 2002 Richard O'Connor Award paper. Arthroscopy 2003;19(3):297–304.

[18] Golish SR, Baumfeld JA, Schoderbek RJ, et al. The effect of femoral tunnel starting position on tunnel length in anterior cruciate ligament reconstruction: a cadaveric study. Arthroscopy 2007, in press.

[19] Morgan CD, Kalman VR, Grawl DM. Definitive landmarks for reproducible tibial tunnel placement in anterior cruciate ligament reconstruction. Arthroscopy 1995;11(3):275–88.

[20] McGuire DA, Wolchok JW. The footprint: a method for checking femoral tunnel placement. Arthroscopy 1998;14(7):777–8.

[21] O'Neill DB. Arthroscopically assisted reconstruction of the anterior cruciate ligament. A follow-up report. J Bone Joint Surg Am 2001;83-A(9):1329–32.

[22] Olszewski AD, Miller MD, Ritchie JR. Ideal tibial tunnel length for endoscopic anterior cruciate ligament reconstruction. Arthroscopy 1998;14(1):9–14.

[23] Miller MD, Olszewski AD. Cruciate ligament graft intra-articular distances. Arthroscopy 1997;13(3):291–5.

[24] Miller MD, Hinkin DT. The "N + 7 rule" for tibial tunnel placement in endoscopic anterior cruciate ligament reconstruction. Arthroscopy 1996;12(1):124–6.

[25] Miller MD, Olszewski AD. Posterior tibial tunnel placement to avoid anterior cruciate ligament graft impingement by the intercondylar roof. An in vitro and in vivo study. Am J Sports Med 1997;25(6):818–22.

[26] Yunes M, Richmond JC, Engels EA, et al. Patellar versus hamstring tendons in anterior cruciate ligament reconstruction: a meta-analysis. Arthroscopy 2001;17(3):248–57.

[27] Ferrari JD, Bach BR Jr. Bone graft procurement for patellar defect grafting in anterior cruciate ligament reconstruction. Arthroscopy 1998;14(5):543–5.

[28] Brand J Jr, Weiler A, Caborn DN, et al. Graft fixation in cruciate ligament reconstruction. Am J Sports Med 2000;28(5):761–74.

[29] Kurosaka M, Yoshiya S, Andrish JT. A biomechanical comparison of different surgical techniques of graft fixation in anterior cruciate ligament reconstruction. Am J Sports Med 1987;15(3):225–9.

[30] Steiner ME, Hecker AT, Brown CH Jr, et al. Anterior cruciate ligament graft fixation. Comparison of hamstring and patellar tendon grafts. Am J Sports Med 1994;22(2):240–6 [discussion: 246–7].

[31] Zantop T, Ruemmler M, Welbers B, et al. Cyclic loading comparison between biodegradable interference screw fixation and biodegradable double cross-pin fixation of human bone-patellar tendon-bone grafts. Arthroscopy 2005;21(8):934–41.

[32] Zantop T, Welbers B, Weimann A, et al. Biomechanical evaluation of a new cross-pin technique for the fixation of different sized bone-patellar tendon-bone grafts. Knee Surg Sports Traumatol Arthrosc 2004;12(6):520–7.

[33] McGuire DA, Barber FA, Elrod BF, et al. Bioabsorbable interference screws for graft fixation in anterior cruciate ligament reconstruction. Arthroscopy 1999;15(5):463–73.

[34] Marti C, Imhoff AB, Bahrs C, et al. Metallic versus bioabsorbable interference screw for fixation of bone-patellar tendon-bone autograft in arthroscopic anterior cruciate ligament reconstruction. A preliminary report. Knee Surg Sports Traumatol Arthrosc 1997;5(4):217–21.

[35] Hackl W, Fink C, Benedetto KP, et al. [Transplant fixation by anterior cruciate ligament reconstruction. Metal vs. bioabsorbable polyglyconate interference screw. A prospective randomized study of 40 patients]. Unfallchirurg 2000;103(6):468–74 [in German].

[36] Abate JA, Fadale PD, Hulstyn MJ, et al. Initial fixation strength of polylactic acid interference screws in anterior cruciate ligament reconstruction. Arthroscopy 1998;14(3):278–84.

[37] Lajtai G, Schmiedhuber G, Unger F, et al. Bone tunnel remodeling at the site of biodegradable interference screws used for anterior cruciate ligament reconstruction: 5-year follow-up. Arthroscopy 2001;17(6):597–602.

[38] Pomeroy G, Baltz M, Pierz K, et al. The effects of bone plug length and screw diameter on the holding strength of bone-tendon-bone grafts. Arthroscopy 1998;14(2):148–52.

[39] Dworsky BD, Jewell BF, Bach BR Jr. Interference screw divergence in endoscopic anterior cruciate ligament reconstruction. Arthroscopy 1996;12(1):45–9.

[40] Pierz K, Baltz M, Fulkerson J. The effect of Kurosaka screw divergence on the holding strength of bone-tendon-bone grafts. Am J Sports Med 1995;23(3):332–5.

[41] Hackl W, Benedetto KP, Hoser C, et al. Is screw divergence in femoral bone-tendon-bone graft fixation avoidable in anterior cruciate ligament reconstruction using a single-incision technique? A radiographically controlled cadaver study. Arthroscopy 2000;16(6):640–7.

[42] Beynnon BD, Johnson RJ, Fleming BC, et al. The measurement of elongation of anterior cruciate-ligament grafts in vivo. J Bone Joint Surg Am 1994;76(4):520–31.

[43] Bylski-Austrow DI, Grood ES, Hefzy MS, et al. Anterior cruciate ligament replacements: a mechanical study of femoral attachment location, flexion angle at tensioning, and initial tension. J Orthop Res 1990;8(4):522–31.

[44] Markolf KL, Burchfield DM, Shapiro MM, et al. Biomechanical consequences of replacement of the anterior cruciate ligament with a patellar ligament allograft. Part I: insertion of the graft and anterior-posterior testing. J Bone Joint Surg Am 1996;78(11):1720–7.

[45] Auge WK 2nd, Yifan K. A technique for resolution of graft-tunnel length mismatch in central third bone-patellar tendon-bone anterior cruciate ligament reconstruction. Arthroscopy 1999;15(8):877–81.

[46] Barber FA. Flipped patellar tendon autograft anterior cruciate ligament reconstruction. Arthroscopy 2000;16(5):483–90.

[47] Sherman OH, Banffy MB. Anterior cruciate ligament reconstruction: which graft is best? Arthroscopy 2004;20(9):974–80.

[48] Goldblatt JP, Fitzsimmons SE, Balk E, et al. Reconstruction of the anterior cruciate ligament: meta-analysis of patellar tendon versus hamstring tendon autograft. Arthroscopy 2005; 21(7):791–803.

[49] Freedman KB, D'Amato MJ, Nedeff DD, et al. Arthroscopic anterior cruciate ligament reconstruction: a metaanalysis comparing patellar tendon and hamstring tendon autografts. Am J Sports Med 2003;31(1):2–11.

[50] Paessler HH, Mastrokalos DS. Anterior cruciate ligament reconstruction using semitendinosus and gracilis tendons, bone patellar tendon, or quadriceps tendon-graft with press-fit fixation without hardware. A new and innovative procedure. Orthop Clin North Am 2003;34(1):49–64.

[51] Weitzel PP, Richmond JC, Altman GH, et al. Future direction of the treatment of ACL ruptures. Orthop Clin North Am 2002;33(4):653–61.

[52] Prodromos CC, Joyce BT, Shi K, et al. A meta-analysis of stability after anterior cruciate ligament reconstruction as a function of hamstring versus patellar tendon graft and fixation type. Arthroscopy 2005;21(10):1202.e1–9.

[53] Ibrahim SA, Al-Kussary IM, Al-Misfer AR, et al. Clinical evaluation of arthroscopically assisted anterior cruciate ligament reconstruction: patellar tendon versus gracilis and semitendinosus autograft. Arthroscopy 2005;21(4):412–7.

[54] Nedeff DD, Bach BR Jr. Arthroscopic anterior cruciate ligament reconstruction using patellar tendon autografts: a comprehensive review of contemporary literature. Am J Knee Surg 2001;14(4):243–58.

[55] Nedeff DD, Bach BR Jr. Arthroscopic anterior cruciate ligament reconstruction using patellar tendon autografts. Orthopedics 2002;25(3):343–57, quiz 358–9.

[56] Buss DD, Min R, Skyhar M, et al. Nonoperative treatment of acute anterior cruciate ligament injuries in a selected group of patients. Am J Sports Med 1995;23(2):160–5.

[57] Shelbourne KD, Trumper RV. Preventing anterior knee pain after anterior cruciate ligament reconstruction. Am J Sports Med 1997;25(1):41–7.

[58] Corry IS, Webb JM, Clingeleffer AJ, et al. Arthroscopic reconstruction of the anterior cruciate ligament. A comparison of patellar tendon autograft and four-strand hamstring tendon autograft. Am J Sports Med 1999;27(4):444–54.

[59] Pinczewski LA, Deehan DJ, Salmon LJ, et al. A five-year comparison of patellar tendon versus four-strand hamstring tendon autograft for arthroscopic reconstruction of the anterior cruciate ligament. Am J Sports Med 2002;30(4):523–36.

[60] Muellner T, Kaltenbrunner W, Nikolic A, et al. Anterior cruciate ligament reconstruction alters the patellar alignment. Arthroscopy 1999;15(2):165–8.

[61] Muellner T, Kaltenbrunner W, Nikolic A, et al. Shortening of the patellar tendon after anterior cruciate ligament reconstruction. Arthroscopy 1998;14(6):592–6.

[62] Adam F, Pape D, Schiel K, et al. Biomechanical properties of patellar and hamstring graft tibial fixation techniques in anterior cruciate ligament reconstruction: experimental study with Roentgen stereometric analysis. Am J Sports Med 2004;32(1):71–8.

[63] Buss DD, Warren RF, Wickiewicz TL, et al. Arthroscopically assisted reconstruction of the anterior cruciate ligament with use of autogenous patellar-ligament grafts. Results after twenty-four to forty-two months. J Bone Joint Surg Am 1993;75(9):1346–55.

[64] Aglietti P, Buzzi R, Zaccherotti G, et al. Patellar tendon versus doubled semitendinosus and gracilis tendons for anterior cruciate ligament reconstruction. Am J Sports Med 1994;22(2): 211–7 [discussion: 217–8].

[65] Maeda A, Shino K, Horibe S, et al. Anterior cruciate ligament reconstruction with multistranded autogenous semitendinosus tendon. Am J Sports Med 1996;24(4):504–9.

[66] Mickelsen PL, Morgan SJ, Johnson WA, et al. Patellar tendon rupture 3 years after anterior cruciate ligament reconstruction with a central one third bone-patellar tendon-bone graft. Arthroscopy 2001;17(6):648–52.

[67] Stein DA, Hunt SA, Rosen JE, et al. The incidence and outcome of patella fractures after anterior cruciate ligament reconstruction. Arthroscopy 2002;18(6):578–83.

[68] Chaudhary D, Monga P, Joshi D, et al. Arthroscopic reconstruction of the anterior cruciate ligament using bone-patellar tendon-bone autograft: experience of the first 100 cases. J Orthop Surg (Hong Kong) 2005;13(2):147–52.

[69] Hiemstra LA, Webber S, MacDonald PB, et al. Knee strength deficits after hamstring tendon and patellar tendon anterior cruciate ligament reconstruction. Med Sci Sports Exerc 2000;32(8):1472–9.

[70] Shelbourne KD, Gray T. Results of anterior cruciate ligament reconstruction based on meniscus and articular cartilage status at the time of surgery. Five- to fifteen-year evaluations. Am J Sports Med 2000;28(4):446–52.

[71] Jomha NM, Pinczewski LA, Clingeleffer A, et al. Arthroscopic reconstruction of the anterior cruciate ligament with patellar-tendon autograft and interference screw fixation. The results at seven years. J Bone Joint Surg Br 1999;81(5):775–9.

[72] Clancy WG Jr, Nelson DA, Reider B, et al. Anterior cruciate ligament reconstruction using one-third of the patellar ligament, augmented by extra-articular tendon transfers. J Bone Joint Surg Am 1982;64(3):352–9.

[73] Jansson KA, Linko E, Sandelin J, et al. A prospective randomized study of patellar versus hamstring tendon autografts for anterior cruciate ligament reconstruction. Am J Sports Med 2003;31(1):12–8.

[74] Aune AK, Holm I, Risberg MA, et al. Four-strand hamstring tendon autograft compared with patellar tendon-bone autograft for anterior cruciate ligament reconstruction. A randomized study with two-year follow-up. Am J Sports Med 2001;29(6):722–8.

[75] Shaieb MD, Kan DM, Chang SK, et al. A prospective randomized comparison of patellar tendon versus semitendinosus and gracilis tendon autografts for anterior cruciate ligament reconstruction. Am J Sports Med 2002;30(2):214–20.

[76] Feller JA, Webster KE. A randomized comparison of patellar tendon and hamstring tendon anterior cruciate ligament reconstruction. Am J Sports Med 2003;31(4):564–73.

[77] Noyes FR, Butler DL, Grood ES, et al. Biomechanical analysis of human ligament grafts used in knee-ligament repairs and reconstructions. J Bone Joint Surg Am 1984;66(3): 344–52.

[78] Woo SL, Hollis JM, Adams DJ, et al. Tensile properties of the human femur-anterior cruciate ligament-tibia complex. The effects of specimen age and orientation. Am J Sports Med 1991;19(3):217–25.

[79] Cooper DE, Deng XH, Burstein AL, et al. The strength of the central third patellar tendon graft. A biomechanical study. Am J Sports Med 1993;21(6):818–24.

[80] Hamner DL, Brown CH Jr, Steiner ME, et al. Hamstring tendon grafts for reconstruction of the anterior cruciate ligament: biomechanical evaluation of the use of multiple strands and tensioning techniques. J Bone Joint Surg Am 1999;81(4):549–57.

[81] Beynnon BD, Johnson RJ, Fleming BC, et al. Anterior cruciate ligament replacement: comparison of bone-patellar tendon-bone grafts with two-strand hamstring grafts. A prospective, randomized study. J Bone Joint Surg Am 2002;84-A(9):1503–13.

[82] Anderson AF, Snyder RB, Lipscomb AB Jr. Anterior cruciate ligament reconstruction. A prospective randomized study of three surgical methods. Am J Sports Med 2001;29(3): 272–9.

Clin Sports Med 26 (2007) 549–565

CLINICS IN SPORTS MEDICINE

ELSEVIER
SAUNDERS

Primary Anterior Cruciate Ligament Reconstruction Using Contralateral Patellar Tendon Autograft

K. Donald Shelbourne, MD*, Bavornrat Vanadurongwan, MD, Tinker Gray, MA

Shelbourne Knee Center at Methodist Hospital, 1815 N. Capitol Avenue, Indianapolis, IN 46202, USA

Anterior cruciate ligament (ACL) reconstruction is a commonly performed procedure, and a number of different grafts for use in ACL reconstruction have been described [1–3]. The autogenous patellar tendon graft seems to be the graft most commonly used for the reconstruction, primarily because of its strength, tight press-fit for early bone-to-bone healing, and early viability [4,5]. Thus, it can respond to the stress of rehabilitation and allows a faster postoperative rehabilitation program than may be possible with other graft choices [6–8]. The main concern about the autogenous patellar tendon graft is related to the morbidity from harvesting approximately one third of the patellar tendon. Possible complications cited by some include quadriceps muscle strength deficit, patellofemoral crepitus, and donor-site anterior knee pain [9,10]; however, some studies have demonstrated that these problems may be related more to poor postoperative rehabilitation than to the graft choice itself [10–12].

Previous studies have reported the results of using the contralateral patellar tendon graft for revision ACL reconstruction [13,14]. The use of the contralateral patellar tendon graft for primary reconstruction was based on observation of the ease with which patients in these studies of revision ACL reconstruction regained full knee range of motion and quadriceps muscle strength in both knees [13,14]. Because of the good results and smooth postoperative rehabilitation, the senior author (KDS) began offering patients the option of using this graft for primary ACL reconstruction in 1994.

RATIONALE FOR USING THE CONTRALATERAL PATELLAR TENDON AUTOGRAFT

The ultimate goal of ACL reconstruction is to restore the injured knee to normal—that is, equal to the contralateral knee. Ideally, the goal is to obtain

*Corresponding author. E-mail address: tgray@aclmd.com (K.D. Shelbourne).

0278-5919/07/$ – see front matter
doi:10.1016/j.csm.2007.06.008

symmetry between knees in range of motion, strength, stability, and function. Rehabilitation after ACL reconstruction involves two different factors. First, rehabilitation for the ACL graft includes obtaining full knee range of motion to stretch the graft to length and not capture the joint. The other goal is to provide the appropriate amount of stress to the ACL graft to stimulate graft maturation but without causing swelling in the joint. Rehabilitation for the graft-donor site, however, is separate and differs from the rehabilitation for the ACL graft. The graft-donor site needs to be stimulated for the patellar tendon to grow in size and in strength. It is advantageous to provide stimulation to the graft-donor site immediately after surgery to take advantage of the inflammatory response from the surgical insult.

When the graft is harvested from the ipsilateral knee, donor site rehabilitation is delayed and is secondary to the goals of rehabilitation for the ACL graft, because the need to regain full range of motion and minimizing swelling takes precedence over other rehabilitation goals. Early aggressive work with quadriceps muscle strengthening exercises to stimulate tendon growth at the graft-donor site causes swelling and decreased range of motion. Therefore, the challenge of rehabilitation using an ipsilateral graft becomes balancing seemingly opposing goals.

With a contralateral autogenous patellar tendon graft, two separate and different rehabilitation programs are implemented for each knee. Early donor-site strengthening can be performed for the contralateral ACL-donor knee to prevent tendon pain and quadriceps muscle weakness. At the same time, rehabilitation for the ACL-reconstructed knee can focus on controlling swelling and soreness and obtaining full range of motion. This approach to surgery and rehabilitation provides the best opportunity to restore the knees to normal and symmetrical condition. Furthermore, it can allow a quicker recovery to activities of daily living and faster return to full capacity in sports activity [15,16].

PREOPERATIVE REHABILITATION

Patients who have an acute ACL injury must undergo rehabilitation before ACL reconstruction. Delaying surgery until preoperative rehabilitation goals are met helps prevent one of the major complications from surgery, loss of knee range of motion [17,18]. The goals of the preoperative rehabilitation program are to regain full knee range of motion, minimize swelling, and obtain good leg control and normal gait. To attain these goals, a cold/compression device (Cryo/Cuff, DonJoy Orthopaedics, Inc., Vista, California) is used to reduce swelling. It is common for patients to have a bent knee after an acute ACL injury. The range of motion in the injured knee should be compared with that in the contralateral normal knee. The authors suggest that knee extension be evaluated with the heel of the foot propped on a bolster to allow the knee to fall into hyperextension, if present. A previous study has shown that 99% of women and 95% of men exhibit some degree of hyperextension in their knees, with averages of 5° and 6°, respectively [19]. Physical therapy exercises for regaining full knee range of motion include a towel-stretch, heel-prop, wall-slide, and heel-slide exercises and gait training.

Once swelling has been controlled and full range of motion has been obtained, patients undergo preoperative stability testing using KT-2000 (MEDmetric Corporation, San Diego, California) arthrometer and isokinetic strength evaluation for both knees. The single-leg hop and single-leg press tests are performed for the uninvolved leg. All preoperative baseline tests are used to provide patients with goals for the return of normal and symmetrical knees following the surgery.

In addition to preparing the knee for surgery, the rehabilitation period is used to prepare the patient mentally for surgery. It allows the patient and family to schedule the surgery at a time that is best for their work and/or school schedules and to concentrate on rehabilitation postoperatively [20]. Appropriate patient education allows the patient to have a good attitude, looking forward to the reconstructive procedure and understanding the rehabilitation process. This delay in surgery does not increase the time it takes an athlete to return to their sport after injury [21] and prevents range-of-motion complications after surgery.

OPERATIVE TECHNIQUE

There are many techniques for ACL reconstructions that involve using different surgical instruments, graft choice, and fixation devices. The authors perform a two-incision miniarthrotomy technique for ACL reconstruction, which has been described in detail elsewhere [22]. This technique allows easy visualization and access to the both ACL footprints and the landmarks that lead to the appropriate tunnels and graft placement. The evidence has shown that an arthrotomy does not slow the rehabilitation [23].

Preoperative Planning with Radiographs

The authors obtain bilateral posteroanterior 45° flexion weight-bearing [24], 60° flexion lateral, and Merchants view [25] radiographs. They measure the intercondylar notch width, patella width, patellar tendon length, and tibial slope. They have found that the width of the patellar tendon is approximately one half the width of the patella. The width of the patellar tendon is an important factor related to strength return after surgery, as explained later. In length the patellar tendon varies from 34 to 74 mm (mean, 49 mm) [22], and the angle of the femoral tunnel can be adjusted to accommodate different lengths of tendon. The width of the intercondylar notch helps the authors plan for the amount of notchplasty needed to accommodate the new 10-mm width of the patellar tendon graft. All these measurements are obtained again intraoperatively.

Femoral Tunnel

The length of the femoral tunnel can be adjusted depending on the length of the graft measured preoperatively. For the longer patellar tendon, the exiting point is more proximal; for the shorter patellar tendon, the exiting point is made more distally. If the pin does not exit in the desired position, it can be redirected using the same starting point. The tunnel is placed as posterior in the notch as possible, and no bone bridge exists between the tunnel and the PCL when seen from the anterior.

The miniarthrotomy technique allows anatomic placement of the femoral tunnel. In this technique, the tunnel can be placed where desired because the anatomic landmarks, such as the intercondylar notch, ACL footprint, and posterior wall, can be seen easily. In addition, the femoral tunnel can be drilled independently of the tibial tunnel. The authors check both tunnel positions by using a straight suction tip, which should pass collinearly through the tibial and femoral tunnel when the knee is flexed 30°. The length of tibial and femoral tunnels and the ACL intra-articular length are measured and recorded.

Graft Harvest

When the patellar tendon graft is harvested from the contralateral knee, several minor changes in surgical routine are made. After the femoral tunnel is drilled, the tourniquet is inflated on the contralateral leg, an incision is made, and the patellar tendon graft is harvested as described. The authors prefer to harvest the graft after the tunnels are prepared so that the graft size can be modified appropriately. The incision begins just medial to the anterior pole of the patella and extends to just below the level of the tibial tubercle. After the patellar tendon (PT) is identified by separating the paratenon and measuring the PT width, a 10-mm-wide bone-patellar tendon-bone graft is harvested from the midportion of the tendon. A previous study has shown that a constant-sized 10-mm central patellar tendon graft can be harvested without compromising ultimate postoperative recovery of quadriceps strength [26]. The bone plugs are approximately 25 mm in length and 10 mm in width. Three drill holes are made in each bone plug, and nonabsorbable sutures (# 2 Ethibond; Ethicon, Somerville, New Jersey) are passed through these holes. The graft then is taken to the back table and prepared by removing excessive bone and fat pad. The harvested site is injected with 0.25% bupivacaine, the knee is wrapped with an elastic bandage, and the tourniquet is deflated.

Fixation with Buttons

The Ethibond sutures placed through the bone plug are passed through the tibial tunnel inside to outside the joint by a suture passer. The bone plug is guided into the tibial tunnel with the cancellous side faced anterior to avoid the impingement of the tendinous part of the graft to the notch. The bone plug is placed at the level of the tibial spine; then the suture ends are passed through the holes of a ligament-fixation button. These ends are tied provisionally with two throws. The sutures in the other bone plug are passed through the femoral tunnel inside the joint to the lateral femoral opening by the suture passer. Pulling these sutures fits the bone plug snugly inside the femoral tunnel, and the tightness of the tendinous part can be palpated inside the joint. The sutures are passed through the ligament fixation button and tied down tightly over the lateral femoral cortex. The sutures on the tibial side are pulled firmly to seat the femoral button. The sutures over the tibial button are retightened at 30° of flexion to make sure the graft is tight enough to provide stability, but the authors make sure they are not too tight to prevent full range of motion in the knee.

After the sutures are tied completely, the knee is moved through its full range of motion equal to the other side. Because the button fixation is not rigid, if the graft is too tight, the slipknots will accommodate by loosening just enough as the knee is moved through its full range of motion. The tightness of the button on the tibia is checked again at 30° of flexion. If it is too loose, the tibial sutures are retied, the knee again is placed through full range of motion, and the button is rechecked for proper tightness. Obtaining full range of motion is the most important goal after surgery; if full range of motion can be achieved with good stability, the patient's goals can be met.

This simple fixation technique has several advantages. Button fixation allows tight bone-to-bone circumferential healing fit without any fixation device in the tunnels. The bone plug in the tibia can be placed at the level of the tibial spine, which provides strong cancellous bone healing. The buttons allow multiple adjustments in graft tension, so that stability is achieved while maintaining full knee range of motion. The results of this surgical technique with button fixation have shown that full range of motion, strength, good function, and stability can be achieved along with an early return to the activity [27,28].

Graft Harvest Site

To prevent permanent patellar and tibial defects caused by harvesting the bone plugs, the bone shavings obtained from drilling the femoral and tibial tunnels are packed into the patellar and tibial defects on the contralateral knee. The patellar tendon defect is closed tightly through the paratenon and patellar tendon so that the patellar tendon defect can be rehabilitated back to normal postoperatively. The graft-donor knee, however, is moved through full range of motion after closure of the tendon to cause the fibers of the patellar tendon to spread out and to ensure that full range of motion can be obtained in the graft-donor knee on the night of surgery.

POSTOPERATIVE REHABILITATION

The clinical outcomes of ACL reconstruction depend on good surgical technique and on rehabilitation. To prevent the morbidity associated with ACL reconstruction, the appropriate rehabilitation program should be done before the surgery and again immediately after surgery. The authors' present philosophy on the rehabilitation of the ACL reconstruction has evolved significantly during past 20 years as they have observed their patients and their results and then adapted their approach to improve final outcomes. They have found that if certain problems are allowed to develop in the early postoperative period, they are difficult to eliminate in the long term. These problems are lack of the full knee extension (compared with the opposite site), hemarthrosis and swelling, and lack of good leg control. Thus, the authors' goals in the early postoperative rehabilitation are (1) to prevent swelling and hemarthrosis; (2) to obtain full extension on the day of surgery; (3) to obtain full flexion as soon as possible after the surgery; and (4) to begin strengthening exercise after symmetric range of motion has been obtained. Using the contralateral patellar tendon graft allows the rehabilitation to be divided between the two knees, needing only to control postoperative swelling, regain full range of motion, and good leg control in the ACL-reconstructed knee and needing only to rehabilitate the graft-source extensor mechanism to return strength and function in the contralateral graft-donor site.

Immediate Postoperative Period

Anterior cruciate ligament–reconstructed knee

The focus of rehabilitation immediately after surgery through the first week is on preventing and limiting a hemarthrosis in the ACL-reconstructed knee while beginning strengthening for the graft-donor site in the contralateral knee. One main way to control a hemarthrosis is for patients to remain at bed rest with the legs elevated above the level of the heart, wearing an antiembolism stocking and a cold/compression device for the first 5 days after surgery. The only time the patient is out of bed during the first 5 days postoperatively is to return home the day after surgery and for bathroom privileges. Patients can perform all the needed exercises while in bed, and the authors do not believe there is any advantage in having patients leave home to attend physical therapy sessions. In fact, they believe that the process of leaving home to attend physical therapy causes the knee to swell, which in turn causes pain and limits range of motion and leg control.

In the operating room a Cryo/Cuff cold/compression device is applied to the ACL-reconstructed knee to prevent a hemarthrosis and swelling. When the patient arrives in the hospital room for the overnight stay after surgery, the ACL-reconstructed leg is placed into a continuous passive motion (CPM) machine set to move the knee from 0° to 30° of flexion. The CPM machine provides gentle motion and also elevates the lower leg above the level of the heart. Ice packs are applied to the graft-donor site, and the leg is propped on a pillow for elevation. With the use of ketorolac infusion for approximately 23 hours postoperatively, continuous cold/compression therapy, and immediate passive knee motion, most patients can perform the rehabilitation exercises without having pain. Patients are instructed to take acetaminophen (1000 mg every 6 hours) beginning immediately when the patient tolerates oral medication. Patients also are instructed to take naproxen (440 mg every 12 hours) once the ketorolac dose is finished. Shelbourne and colleagues [29] found that with this pain-management protocol patients took, on average, 1.9 doses propoxyphene (65 mg) per day during the first week after surgery.

Patients begin knee range-of-motion exercises when they arrive in the hospital room after recovery. The heel-prop exercise is done by propping both legs into extension with the heels resting on the bolster, allowing for any hyperextension. The bolster should be high enough to elevate the calf and thigh off the level of the bed (Fig. 1). A small 2.5-pound weight may be placed just distal to the incision on the ACL-reconstructed knee for more extension. A towel-stretch exercise is performed using a towel looped around the midfoot to bring the knee into hyperextension (Fig. 2). An active heel-lift exercise can be combined

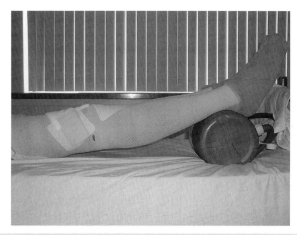

Fig. 1. Heel-prop exercise. Both heels are propped on a bolster so the calf and thigh are elevated off the bed enough to allow the knees to fall into hyperextension.

with the towel stretch to achieve good quadriceps control by trying to keep the heel of the affected leg elevated without the use of the towel to hold it for 5 seconds. Five to 10 towel-extension exercises are performed on each leg daily to maintain full extension. A straight leg-raising exercise also is performed for good leg control.

For the flexion exercise, the CPM machine is progressed to 125° and held in this position for about 1 minute. This exercise is done slowly and as tolerated by the patient four times per day. Heel slides also are performed for both the ACL-reconstructed knee and the contralateral graft-donor knee. The terminal

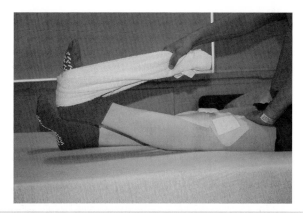

Fig. 2. Towel-stretch exercise. A towel is looped around the midfoot, and the patient holds the ends of the towel. The patient places one hand just above the knee and uses the other hand to pull the towel toward them, which brings the knee into hyperextension.

flexion is held for 1 minute, and the number of centimeters that the heel has moved is recorded. The authors have found that the use of a measuring stick to measure flexion is a useful tool for patients to monitor their progress (Fig. 3). The zero end of the stick is placed at the heel, and the patient can bend the knee and see how many centimeters the heel has moved. This method is easier for patients than trying to determine the degree of flexion in the knee. Having a number makes it easy for the patient to communicate with the doctor or physical therapist regarding progress. In the ACL-reconstructed knee, flexion should be 120° to 130° immediately postoperatively or about 10° less than the full flexion achieved in the opposite graft-donor knee.

Following these exercises, the Cryo/Cuff is applied to the ACL-reconstructed knee, and the leg is placed back into the CPM set from 0° to 30° of flexion. The water for the cold/compression devise is changed once every waking hour to control pain and swelling. The patient is allowed to ambulate with full weight bearing as tolerated; a patient who is unsteady or at risk of falling can use crutches or a walker.

Graft-donor knee

The graft-donor knee does not have an effusion after surgery because harvesting the graft is an extra-articular procedure; however, ice packs are applied frequently for pain control. In addition, the authors place a subcutaneous Constavac drain (Stryker Medical, Kalamazoo, Michigan) in the knee. Full range of motion can be obtained on the day of surgery; thus, graft-donor site rehabilitation exercise can begin immediately. Within 2 hours after surgery, patients begin exercises to stimulate the regrowth of the patellar tendon by using a small leg-press machine (The Shuttle, Contemporary Design Company, Glacier, WA) that is lightweight and portable and applies light resistance (Fig. 4). Resistance is

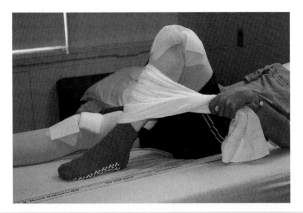

Fig. 3. Heel slide with towel. The patient loops the towel around the front of the shin and pulls on the end of the towel to assist with knee flexion. A yardstick is used to monitor progress in knee flexion. The zero end of the yardstick is placed at the heel, and the patient can record the number of centimeters the heel moves.

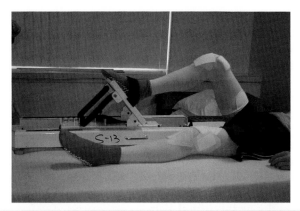

Fig. 4. Shuttle machine. The Shuttle is a small leg-press unit that the patient uses to perform high-repetition and low-resistance exercise to stimulate regrowth of the patellar tendon.

provided by the placement of the rubber cords, each adding additional resistance. Using all six cords can create 14 kg of resistance. The patient is instructed to use the amount of resistance that allows them to start with 25 repetitions. Patients perform this exercise four to five times each day, progressing toward 100 repetitions during one session. During this strengthening program, if flexion in the graft-donor site starts to decrease (as measured daily by the yard stick), the patient is advised either to decrease the Shuttle exercise resistance, the frequency, or both until full flexion returns.

Home instructions
Patients are released from the hospital the day after surgery after they have shown that they understand the exercises to be performed. Patients are instructed to remain at bed rest except for bathroom privileges and to return to the clinic for evaluation 5 days after surgery. The physical therapist calls the patient daily at home to check on progress and to answer any questions the patient might have.

Early Postoperative Period
Anterior cruciate ligament–reconstructed knee
Patients return for evaluation by the physician and physical therapist about 5 days after surgery, which is past the time of the initial inflammatory response from surgery. For the first month after surgery, the emphasis of rehabilitation for the ACL-reconstructed knee is on controlling swelling, maintaining full hyperextension in the knee, and obtaining full knee flexion that is symmetrical to the contralateral knee. In addition, the normal gait pattern is emphasized along with certain daily habits in standing and sitting that will foster maintaining full knee range of motion.

Each patient should be able to perform a straight leg raise without a lag and to perform an active heel lift with the knee hyperextension while the thigh lies on the table. Whenever sitting, the patient should be performing a heel-prop exercise. Whenever the patient is standing, the weight should be shifted to the ACL-reconstructed leg with the knee locked in hyperextension (Fig. 5). Towel-stretch exercises also continue in this phase to maintain the full extension.

Use of the CPM machine is discontinued, but the heel-slide and the wall-slide exercises are still done routinely for flexion exercise. All range-of-motion exercises are performed two to four times per day. The cold/compression device is used by the patient as needed throughout the day to control swelling, and continued use throughout the night is encouraged. By the end of the second week, patients usually report that they are performing their full normal activities of daily living (having returned to school or work). If excessive effusion occurs during this period, patients are instructed to use the cold/compression device with elevation frequently during the day and to decrease daily activities.

Graft-donor knee
The ACL graft-donor knee should have full extension and flexion easily. The exercises with the Shuttle machine continue during the second week postoperatively, and the patient should progress until he or she can perform the maximum number of repetitions with the greatest possible resistance. In this

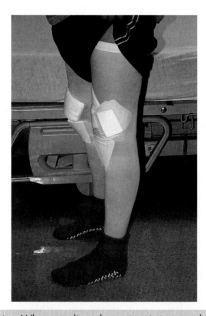

Fig. 5. Standing exercise. When standing, the patient is instructed to shift weight onto the ACL-reconstructed knee and to stand with the knee in full extension as a means of fostering good leg control and of avoiding favoring that leg.

period, the focus remains on high-repetition/low-resistance exercise to stimulate the harvested site and increase the size of the patellar tendon.

The patient is given a step box so that step exercise can be done using the graft-donor knee to stimulate patellar tendon regrowth. The step box is a hinged, foldable device. The height of the step box can be adjusted adjustable from 2 to 8 inches off the floor for increasing difficulty. Forward step-down exercises are prescribed (Fig. 6), and patients are encouraged to use good technique. The patient is instructed to do 25 to 100 repetitions three to four times per day at the selected height. If patient cannot do 25 repetitions, the height of the step box should be lowered. When the patient is able to do 100 repetitions, the height of the step box is raised.

Weight-training exercises, such as single leg-press and single leg-extension exercises, can be added once the patient can easily do sets of 100 step-downs several times per day and for some patients can begin as early as 2 weeks to 1 month after surgery. Each exercise is performed only on the graft-donor leg, because in the ACL-reconstructed knee the focus is only on controlling swelling and on range of motion . Typically, the patient is instructed to start with the half of their body weight or less for the leg-press machine and 2 to 5 lbs with the leg-extension exercise. Three to five sessions per day of 25 repetitions of each exercise usually are sufficient. When patients are able to do all the repetitions easily, they can increase the amount of weight used for the exercise. If the patient develops soreness that persists and is not decreased with cryotherapy, he or she is advised to decrease the exercise weight, the frequency, or both.

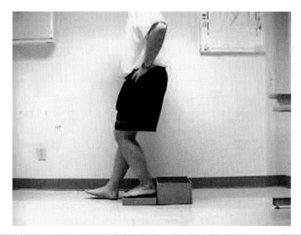

Fig. 6. Step-down exercise. The patient stands on the step box, on the graft-donor leg, so that the ACL-reconstructed leg is free to be lowered to the front of the box. The shoulders should be level over the hips, and the graft-donor knee should bend so that other foot barely touches the floor. The patient should straighten the graft-donor knee while keeping the shoulders and hips level. The step exercises should be done under slow control to make sure that the quadriceps muscles are being contracted.

Strengthening Period

The goal is for patients to be able to sit comfortably on their heels with their ankles in plantarflexion before beginning bilateral strengthening exercises. Some patients can begin this phase of rehabilitation as early as 1 month post-operatively. Stationary bicycling, stair-climbing exercise, or an elliptical trainer can be used, depending on what is available to the patient. These activities must be started very slowly and cautiously, with monitoring of the amount of swelling in the ACL-reconstructed knee.

The ability to return to activities depends on the strength of the graft-donor knee, the presence of full motion in both knees, and the absence of an effusion in the ACL-reconstructed knee. The isokinetic strength test and KT 1000 arthrometer test are performed monthly to monitor stability and strength progress. When the difference in quadriceps muscle strength between knees is less than 10%, the patient can begin bilateral weight-strengthening exercises. Until then, the patient continues to perform single-leg weight training in the graft-donor knee until the legs have nearly symmetrical strength. The timing of strength return varies greatly among patients, and the exercises for strength must be prescribed individually according to the rehabilitation goals.

Patients can begin to perform agility drills to increase proprioception. Straight-line, forward, and backward jogging, as well as lateral sides and crossovers, can be done. Noncompetitive sport-specific drills can be performed as tolerated. The addition of sport-specific drills helps motivate patients, but patients are warned that if they lose any range of motion in the knee or it becomes swollen, the activities must be decreased accordingly.

Return to Competition

There is no strict guideline or an absolute number of weeks or months after surgery that patients can return to competition. Determining the exact time when patients return to activities is difficult, because progress is a gradual and highly individual development and is related to the patient's particular sport. The authors' guideline is for patients to have equal range motion and equal strength in both knees before they begin to play. They believe that once the symmetry is achieved between the knees, the level of activities can increase slowly, starting from an individual noncompetitive activity and progressing to the sport activity at the patient's previous competitive level.

For competitive athletes who have achieved the goals of symmetric range of motion and strength, the authors recommend that they train hard every other day as they begin the sport-specific training. The authors have observed that it is difficult for athletes to perform their sport at half-speed and be able to compete well in practice, so they tend to practice hard once they feel comfortable enough to do so, even when they are told to practice at reduced intensity. After the training day, the ACL-reconstructed knee may have swelling and decreased knee flexion, and the graft-donor knee may have patellar tendon soreness. The athletes need a day of rest between the hard training days. This way, when the athlete is practicing, he or she can perform as expected but then take a day off to let the knees recover. Gradually, the athlete will condition the knees to feel comfortable enough to practice 2 consecutive days and then need a day off and finally be able to practice and compete all the time. Good communication is required between the physician, physical therapist, patient, and coach for this plan of recovery to sports to be successful. Although competitive athletes can get back to practice around 2 months postoperatively and back to competition around 4 months postoperatively, an additional 2 months of playing are needed before the athlete feels normal again.

Time-restricted protocols for ACL rehabilitation have been used because of concern about reinjury of the ACL-reconstructed knee. The authors have found that the time after surgery before return to sports has not been a factor for reinjury. Instead, not having symmetrical knees for strength and range of motion has been more of a factor for reinjury.

RESULTS OF USING THE CONTRALATERAL PATELLAR TENDON GRAFT

Only a few studies have investigated the use of a patellar tendon graft from the contralateral knee for primary ACL reconstruction [15,30,31]. Shelbourne and Urch [15] were the first to describe their experience in patients who underwent surgery between 1994 and 1997. Their study compared the results of 434 patients who underwent surgery with a graft from the contralateral knee with the results of 228 patients who underwent surgery with a graft from the ipsilateral knee. The study showed that patients in the contralateral group had statistically significantly more knee flexion than the ipsilateral group at 1 and 2 weeks after surgery. Similarly, patients in the contralateral group had statistically significantly greater quadriceps muscle strength in the ACL-reconstructed knee than patients in the ipsilateral group at 1, 2, and 4 months postoperatively and in graft-donor knee at 1 and 2 months postoperatively. For the patients in the competitive subgroup, the mean time to full sports participation was 4.1 months in those who had a contralateral graft and 5.5 months in those who had an ipsilateral graft. There was no difference in knee stability, as measured objectively with the KT-1000 (MEDmetric Corporation, San Diego, California) arthrometer, at follow-up [15].

Mastrokalos and colleagues [30] performed a similar study to compare donor-site morbidity in patients who received ipsilateral (52 patients) or contralateral (48 patients) patellar tendon grafts. Donor-site morbidity was evaluated by comparing results reported for the graft-donor site in each group with the results reported for the ACL-reconstructed knee in the contralateral group. They found no difference between groups in stability scores, Cincinnati or Tegner subjective scores, or numbness at the incision site. They found that the graft knee had more local tenderness for both the ipsilateral group and the graft-donor knee in the contralateral group than the ACL-reconstructed knee in the contralateral group. These groups also had greater kneeling pain and knee-walking pain than was reported for the ACL-reconstructed knee in the contralateral group. Mastrokalos and colleagues [30] reported that the mean time to return to activities of daily living was 5.2 weeks in the ipsilateral group and 4.9 weeks in the contralateral group. The mean time to return to unrestricted athletic activity was 7.4 months in the contralateral group and 7.8 months in the ipsilateral group; however, the rehabilitation program specifically restricted patients from returning to unrestricted athletic activity until 6 months postoperatively. The authors concluded that there was no advantage in using the contralateral graft over the ipsilateral graft because the symptoms related to donor-site morbidity are shifted from the injured knee to the healthy knee. The rehabilitation program, however, did not describe any specific rehabilitation for the graft-donor knee that was different from that for the ipsilateral knee or that was specific for regaining strength and size [30].

Zink and colleagues [31] evaluated strength recovery after ACL reconstruction with a contralateral graft to determine if there were any gender differences. The study group included 102 patients, and the investigators tested quadriceps and hamstring muscle strength using both isokinetic testing and leg-press testing. The only difference in strength was that men had better hamstring muscle strength than women at 5 weeks, 10 weeks, and 4 months postoperatively, but there was no difference at 6 months postoperatively. The difference in hamstring muscle strength between the involved and uninvolved legs before surgery was 89% for women and 96% for men, but there was no mention as to whether this difference was statistically significant [31]. It is possible that the preoperative hamstring strength deficit for women affected the return of strength postoperatively.

DISCUSSION

The specific rehabilitation as described for the graft-donor site and ACL-reconstructed knees needs to be done precisely to realize the advantages of the return of strength and range of motion. If a contralateral graft is used, and rehabilitation is not followed, patients undoubtedly will be unsatisfied with the results.

In certain situations the contralateral graft can be extremely helpful for primary ACL reconstruction: (1) in patients who have poor quadriceps muscle strength in the involved leg; (2) in patients who have small patellar tendons; (3) in patients who have difficultly reducing their swelling and obtaining full range of motion after an acute injury; and (4) in patients who want to return to normal, everyday activities as soon as possible.

Patients who have significant strength deficits either from an acute injury or from chronic instability have a better chance of achieving full symmetrical strength after surgery when a contralateral graft is used than when an ipsilateral graft is used on an already weakened leg. In a group of patients who had ACL reconstruction with an ipsilateral graft, Shelbourne and Johnson [32] found that patients in whom quadriceps muscle strength of the involved leg was less than 75% of the strength of the noninvolved leg before surgery had significantly less strength at all time periods after surgery than patients whose weaker leg had more than 90% of the strength in the contralateral leg before surgery. The mean strength in the involved knee at 2 years postoperatively was 91% in the group with poor preoperative strength and 96% in the group with good strength.

In the same study Shelbourne and Johnson [32] also evaluated the effect of patellar tendon size on the return of strength after surgery. Patients who had a small tendon ($\leq$ 26 mm wide) had significantly less strength after surgery than patients who had medium (27–30 mm) or wide (31–36 mm) tendons until 2 years postoperatively. Thus, for a patient who has a small patellar tendon and significant quadriceps muscle strength loss, the contralateral graft is an ideal choice.

Some patients struggle to achieve all the preoperative goals of surgery, especially to obtain full knee range of motion and reduce swelling. In the authors' experience, patients who have difficulty achieving these goals before surgery also have difficulty after surgery. The use of the contralateral graft allows these patients to focus only on reducing swelling and obtaining full range of motion in the ACL-reconstructed knee without the concern of working on strength in the same leg.

Although the use of the contralateral graft is thought to be most advantageous for athletes who desire or need to return to sports quickly, it also is advantageous for people who want to return quickly and comfortably to the everyday activities at home, work, and school. Patients are able to achieve normal knee motion in both legs and to walk with a normal gait quickly after surgery. Patients cannot favor one leg over another, because both have undergone surgery. The rehabilitation coupled with performing everyday activities of walking, squatting, and climbing stairs without favoring one side forces patients to use both legs normally, which the authors believe fosters the return of normal strength. Therefore, patients who have an immediate need to perform everyday activities can do so quickly and then return to other sporting activities on a relaxed time schedule.

SUMMARY

The autogenous patellar tendon graft is an excellent graft choice for use in ACL reconstruction, and the reported problems associated with its use are related primarily to rehabilitation issues. With the contralateral patellar tendon graft, the goals of rehabilitation program can be divided between the knees. These principles of the rehabilitation should be taken seriously for the best opportunity to restore symmetrical knees and more predictable results without complications.

References

[1] Miller SL, Gladstone JN. Graft selection in anterior cruciate ligament reconstruction. Orthop Clin North Am 2002;33:675–83.

[2] Petrigliano FA, McAllister DR, Wu BM. Tissue engineering for anterior cruciate ligament reconstruction: a review of current strategies. Arthroscopy 2006;22:441–51.

[3] West RV, Harner CD. Graft selection in anterior cruciate ligament reconstruction. J Am Acad Orthop Surg 2005;13:197–207.

[4] Rougraff B, Shelbourne KD. Arthroscopic and histologic analysis of human patellar tendon autografts used for anterior cruciate ligament reconstruction. Am J Sports Med 1993;21:277–84.

[5] Rougraff BT, Shelbourne KD. Early histologic appearance of human patellar tendon auto-grafts used for anterior cruciate ligament reconstruction. Knee Surg Sports Traumatol Arthrosc 1999;7:9–14.

[6] Aglietti P, Buzzi R, Zaccherotti G, et al. Patellar tendon versus doubled semitendinosus and gracilis tendons for anterior cruciate ligament reconstruction. Am J Sports Med 1994;22: 2–11.

[7] Beynnon BD, Johnson RJ, Fleming BC, et al. Anterior cruciate ligament replacement: comparison of bone-patellar tendon-bone graft with two-strand hamstrings grafts. A prospective randomized study. J Bone Joint Surg Am 2002;84:1503–12.

[8] Shelton WR, Papendick L, Dukes AD. Autograft versus allograft anterior cruciate ligament reconstruction. Arthroscopy 1997;13:446–69.

[9] Freedman KB, D'Amato MJ, Nedeff DD, et al. Arthroscopic anterior cruciate ligament reconstruction: a metaanalysis comparing patellar tendon and hamstring tendon autografts. Am J Sports Med 2003;31:2–11.

[10] Kartus J, Magnusson L, Stener S, et al. Complications following arthroscopic anterior cruciate ligament reconstruction. A 2-5-year follow-up of 604 patients with special emphasis on anterior knee pain. Knee Surg Sports Traumatol Arthrosc 1999;7:2–8.

[11] Sachs RA, Daniel DM, Stone ML, et al. Patellofemoral problems after anterior cruciate ligament reconstruction. Am J Sports Med 1989;17:760–5.

[12] Shelbourne KD, Nitz P. Accelerated rehabilitation after anterior cruciate ligament reconstruction. Am J Sports Med 1990;18:292–9.

[13] Rubinstein RA, Shelbourne KD, VanMeter CD, et al. Isolated autogenous bone-patellar tendon-bone graft site morbidity. Am J Sports Med 1994;22:324–7.

[14] Shelbourne KD, O'Shea JJ. Revision anterior cruciate ligament reconstruction using contra-lateral bone patellar tendon bone graft. Instr Course Lect 2002;51:343–6.

[15] Jari S, Shelbourne KD. Staged bilateral anterior cruciate ligament reconstruction with use of contralateral patellar tendon autograft. Am J Sports Med 2002;30:437–40.

[16] Shelbourne KD, Urch SE. Primary anterior cruciate ligament reconstruction using the contra-lateral autogenous patellar tendon. Am J Sports Med 2000;28:651–8.

[17] Mohtadi NG, Webster-Bogaert SW, Fowler PJ. Limitation of motion following anterior ligament reconstruction. A case control study. Am J Sports Med 1991;19:620–5.

[18] Shelbourne KD, Wilckens JH, Mollabashy A, et al. Arthrofibrosis in acute anterior cruciate ligament reconstruction. The effect of timing of reconstruction and rehabilitation. Am J Sports Med 1991;19:332–6.

[19] DeCarlo MS, Sell K. Normative data for range of motion and single leg hop in high school athletes. J Sports Rehab 1997;6:246–55.

[20] Udry E, Shelbourne KD, Gray T. Psychological readiness for ACL surgery: describing and comparing the adolescent and adult experience. J Athletic Training 2003;38:167–71.

[21] Shelbourne KD, Foulk DA. Timing of surgery in anterior cruciate ligament tears on the return of quadriceps muscle strength after reconstruction using an autogenous patellar tendon graft. Am J Sports Med 1995;23:686–9.

[22] Shelbourne KD. Mini-open ACL reconstruction using contralateral patellar tendon. Techniques in Orthopaedics 2005;20:353–60.

[23] Shelbourne KD, Rettig AC, Hardin G, et al. Miniarthrotomy versus arthroscopic-assisted anterior cruciate ligament reconstruction with autogenous patellar tendon graft. Arthroscopy 1993;9:72–5.

[24] Rosenberg TD, Paulos LE, Parker RD, et al. The forty-five degree posterior flexion weight-bearing radiograph of the knee. J Bone Joint Surg Am 1988;70:1479–83.

[25] Merchant AC, Mercer RL, Jacobsen RH, et al. Roentgenographic analysis of patellofemoral congruence. J Bone Joint Surg 1974;56A:1391–6.

[26] Shelbourne KD, Rubinstein RA, VanMeter CD, et al. Correlation of remaining patellar tendon width with quadriceps strength after autogenous bone-patellar tendon-bone anterior cruciate ligament reconstruction. Am J Sports Med 1994;22:774–8.

[27] Shelbourne KD, Gray T. Anterior cruciate ligament reconstruction with autogenous patellar tendon graft followed by accelerated rehabilitation. A two-to nine-year followup. Am J Sports Med 1997;25:786–95.

[28] Shelbourne KD, Gray T. Results of anterior cruciate ligament reconstruction based on the meniscal and articular cartilage status at the time of surgery: five- to fifteen-year evaluations. Am J Sports Med 2000;28:446–52.

[29] Shelbourne KD, Liotta FJ, Goodloe SL. Preemptive pain management program for anterior cruciate ligament reconstruction. Am J Knee Surg 1998;11:116–9.

[30] Mastrokalos DS, Springer J, Siebold R, et al. Donor site morbidity and return to the preinjury activity level after anterior cruciate ligament reconstruction using ipsilateral and contralateral patellar tendon autograft. A retrospective, nonrandomized study. Am J Sports Med 2005;33:85–93.

[31] Zink EJ, Trumper RV, Smidt CR, et al. Gender comparison of knee strength recovery following ACL reconstruction with contralateral patellar tendon graft. Biomed Sci Instrum 2005;41:323–8.

[32] Shelbourne KD, Johnson BC. Effects of patellar tendon width and preoperative quadriceps strength on strength return after anterior cruciate ligament reconstruction with ipsilateral bone-patellar tendon-bone autograft. Am J Sports Med 2004;32:1474–8.

Clin Sports Med 26 (2007) 567–585

CLINICS IN SPORTS MEDICINE

ELSEVIER
SAUNDERS

Principles for Using Hamstring Tendons for Anterior Cruciate Ligament Reconstruction

Keith W. Lawhorn, MD[a,b,*], Stephen M. Howell, MD[c]

[a]Uniformed Services University of the Health Sciences, 4301 Jones Bridge Road, Bethesda, MD 20814, USA
[b]Advanced Orthopaedics and Sports Medicine Institute, 3700 Joseph Siewick Drive, Suite 205, Fairfax VA 22033, USA
[c]Department of Mechanical and Aeronautical Engineering, University of California Davis, Davis, CA, USA

HISTORY

Hamstring tendons continue to gain in popularity as a graft source for anterior cruciate ligament (ACL) reconstruction. The excellent biomechanical properties of the double-looped hamstring (DLHS) graft, low harvest morbidity, improved fixation, and multiple level I and level II evidence from clinical studies demonstrating outcomes equal to those obtained with other autogenous graft sources used for ACL reconstruction provide numerous reasons for this gain in popularity [1–6]. Previous clinical outcome studies showing that knees with hamstring grafts were inferior to knees with bone-patella tendon-bone (BPTB) graft ACL reconstruction might have resulted from poor fixation and the use of single-bundle or single-looped graft constructs. Several biomechanical studies have shown that the DLHS graft is two times stronger and stiffer than a 10-mm autogenous BPTB graft [7,8]. With the advent of newer fixation devices designed specifically for the DLHS graft and with tunnel placement techniques designed to prevent graft impingement, functional outcomes and stability using autograft hamstring tendons have been improved. No study to date demonstrates a superiority of any graft source for ACL reconstruction in terms of stability and functional outcomes, but many believe that the morbidity of hamstring graft harvest is less than the morbidity of BPTB harvest [6,9,10]. The incidence of anterior knee pain, knee extension loss, kneeling pain, and arthritis have been demonstrated to be statistically greater with BPTB grafts than with DLHS grafts used for ACL reconstruction [3,11]. A recent prospective study of two groups equally matched in demographics,

*Corresponding author. 3700 Joseph Siewick Dr., Suite 205, Fairfax, VA 22033.
E-mail address: klawhorn@cox.net (K.W. Lawhorn).

0278-5919/07/$ – see front matter
doi:10.1016/j.csm.2007.07.002
sportsmed.theclinics.com

meniscal tears, and cartilage injury and with a minimum 5-year follow-up demonstrated a statistically higher incidence of osteoarthritis of the knee in patients who had a BPTB graft (50%) than in patients who had a DLHS graft (17%) for ACL reconstruction [3]. The study found no differences in stability and functional outcomes between the two groups. It remains unknown if longer follow-up of patients who have had DLHS ACL reconstruction will demonstrate an incidence of osteoarthritic changes similar to that seen in patients who have BPTB autografts. Nonetheless, autograft hamstring tendons remain an excellent graft source for ACL reconstruction while minimizing graft-harvest morbidity.

OVERVIEW OF STRUCTURAL PROPERTIES OF FIXATION DEVICES

Despite the excellent biomechanical properties of autogenous hamstring tendons and the low morbidity associated with hamstring harvest, sound fixation of soft tissue grafts for ACL reconstruction is paramount to ensure good stability and functional outcomes. Fixation devices should resist slippage under cyclical load, provide high stiffness and high strength, and promote biologic healing of the graft to the tunnel wall so that aggressive rehabilitation can be initiated safely. The healing of a soft tissue graft to a bone tunnel takes longer than the healing of a bone-plug graft [12]. Therefore, soft tissue graft-fixation devices must maintain their structural properties for resistance to slippage, stiffness, and strength for longer periods of time, because the hamstring graft and the fixation together function as the ACL until a secure attachment is formed between the graft and bone. Surgeons need to know the structural properties of both tibial and femoral soft tissue fixation devices available to determine the optimum fixation of a soft tissue graft and ensure excellent outcomes.

Tibial Fixation

The weakest biomechanical link of any ACL reconstruction is the tibial fixation. Therefore the device used for tibial fixation is the more important fixation device and determines the properties of a soft tissue ACL construct. The WasherLoc (Arthrotek/Biomet, Warsaw, Indiana), interference screws, Intrafix (Depuy Mitek, Raynham, Massachusetts), CentraLoc (Arthrotek/Biomet, Warsaw, Indiana), bone staples, and suture posts have all been used for tibial soft tissue graft fixation. The authors prefer to use the WasherLoc device exclusively for tibial fixation, based on biomechanical testing and clinical outcomes. The WasherLoc is a screw and washer device designed to achieve distal intratunnel fixation using lag screw fixation to cortical bone. The distal intratunnel position gives the screw and washer a low profile, thereby significantly reducing the need for hardware removal because of prominence. The 13 tines of the washer penetrate the tendon graft, and the lag screw compresses the washer and graft against the corticocancellous bone of the posterior wall of the tibial tunnel. The WasherLoc hamstring graft construct has high strength (905 newtons [N]), stiffness (248 N/mm), and resistance to graft slippage under cyclical load conditions when tested in human cadaveric bone [13]. The WasherLoc fixation of a DLHS graft is the only tibial fixation device that approximates the biomechanical properties of the native ACL when tested in human bone [14]. In addition, when tested in an in vivo animal model, WasherLoc fixation of a soft tissue graft maintains its biomechanical properties over time and promotes biologic healing of the graft–bone tunnel interface, a stark contrast to interference screw fixation of a soft tissue graft [15]. Another advantage of the WasherLoc is that the device allows bone grafting of the tibial tunnel, which eliminates voids, increases stiffness, enhances tendon–bone tunnel healing, and prevents tunnel widening [16–18]. Finally, the structural properties of the WasherLoc and its performance in vivo ensure safe use of aggressive rehabilitation and an early return to sports at 4 months with high clinical success [19].

Femoral Fixation

Numerous femoral fixation devices designed specifically for hamstring ACL reconstruction exist for soft tissue ACL graft fixation. Cross-pin devices such as the EZLoc (Arthrotek/Biomet, Warsaw, Indiana), Bone Mulch Screw (Arthrotek/Biomet, Warsaw, Indiana), RigidFix (Depuy Mitek, Raynham, Massachusetts), and Transfix (Arthrex, Naples, Florida) devices afford better ultimate tensile failure load and stiffness data than other types of femoral fixation such interference screw fixation, EndoButton (Smith and Nephew; Andover, Massachusetts), and suture posts. For femoral fixation, the authors prefer the EZLoc fixation device because of the device's biomechanical properties and its ease of use. The EZLoc provides high strength and stiffness fixation with minimal slippage under cyclical loading conditions. The strength of the EZLoc is greater than 1400 N tested on the bench top. The stiffness of the EZLoc implant fixed in human bone is high because the device is seated directly against cortical bone. The slippage of the implant and graft therefore should be negligible, because the graft is looped directly over the cross-pin of the device, avoiding the use of any linkage material. Avoiding the use of linkage material improves the stiffness of fixation while minimizing graft motion in the bone tunnel during biologic healing to the tunnel wall. The properties of the EZLoc device allow the safe use of an aggressive rehabilitation protocol. The EZLoc also affords the surgeon the ability to confirm 100% graft capture by the fixation device. The graft is passed through the cross-pin loop of the EZLoc outside the patient before tunnel graft passage. With other cross-pin devices such as the RigidFix and Transfix, "blind" graft passage and fixation must be performed with no guarantee of complete graft capture and with the added possibility of graft laceration and damage [20]. Without complete graft capture or with graft damage, the functional cross-sectional area of the graft tissue is diminished, resulting in a weaker graft fixation construct. The EZLoc also allows the surgeon to tension all four bundles of a soft tissue graft equally. Because the grafts are pulled individually over the cross-pin, all graft bundles can be tensioned equally, maximizing the properties of the graft tissue. Finally, the EZLoc can help promote the biologic healing of a soft tissue graft to the bone tunnel by allowing a snug fit of the graft in the bony tunnel. The EZLoc allows sizing of the graft and femoral tunnel so that the snugness of fit can be optimized at the time of graft sizing.

TUNNEL PLACEMENT

Precise tunnel placement is the single most important technical issue associated with outcomes of ACL reconstruction. No graft source, fixation, or rehabilitation protocol can overcome the complications associated with poor tunnel placement. Poor tunnel placement can lead to roof impingement, posterior cruciate ligament (PCL) impingement, and abnormal tensile graft forces. Complications of impingement lead to loss of knee motion with increased graft laxity and instability. The best treatment for avoiding complications associated with impingement is prevention.

Numerous tunnel techniques exist for femoral and tibial tunnel placement for ACL reconstruction. Transtibial, transportal, and two-incision techniques are used for tunnel placement, and successful outcomes have been documented for each. Tunnel placement, however, is more exacting for a hamstring graft because the intra-articular cross-sectional area of collagen is greater for a hamstring graft than for a BPTB graft. It also is important for surgeons to realize that the anatomy of graft sources cannot duplicate the native anatomic insertion site of the ACL; surgeons can, however, duplicate the anatomic intra-articular ACL position with the ACL graft. The authors prefer the transtibial technique for tunnel preparation, using a tibial guide (65° guide, Arthrotek, Warsaw, Indiana) that references the bone of the intercondylar roof with the knee in full extension and the use of size-specific femoral aimers through the tibial tunnel for femoral tunnel positioning. The 65° guide seats in the intercondylar notch with the knee in full extension. The guide takes into account the variability of intercondylar roof angles and knee extension that exists in individual patients, enabling surgeons to customize the position of the ACL graft for any given patient. The 65° guide therefore serves to position the ACL graft posterior and parallel to the intercondylar roof when the knee is in full extension, duplicating the anatomic position of the native ACL. Multiple studies have demonstrated the validity and reliability of tibial tunnel placement within the native ACL tibial footprint while positioning the graft posterior and parallel to the intercondylar roof and avoiding roof impingement [21,22]. Roof impingement is the result of too anterior a position of the tibial tunnel leading to an error in sagittal-plane positioning of the tibial tunnel. Roof impingement leads to increased knee laxity, graft failure, knee effusions, anterior knee pain with attempted terminal extension, and flexion contractures [23,24].

With the transtibial tunnel technique, surgeons focus on precise positioning of one tunnel: the tibial tunnel. Surgeons then rely on the position of the tibial tunnel in the sagittal and coronal planes to help determine the position of the femoral tunnel. Thus, the critical tunnel is the tibial tunnel. The position of the femoral tunnel in the sagittal and coronal planes determines tensile graft behavior and is essentially automatic once the tibial tunnel is positioned properly. Posterior femoral tunnel placement in the sagittal plane is achieved consistently using size-specific femoral aimers through the tibial tunnel. With the transtibial tunnel technique, the tibial tunnel must be positioned between the tibial spines at an angle of 60° to 65° in the coronal plane to establish tensile graft behavior similar to that of the native ACL and to avoid PCL impingement [25]. An error in coronal plane positioning of the tibial tunnel thus leads to an error in coronal-plane positioning of the femoral tunnel, because little change can be made in the coronal plane when positioning the femoral tunnel using the tibial tunnel. The 65° guide includes a coronal alignment rod to increase the accuracy of tibial tunnel positioning in the coronal plane [26]. Tibial tunnels positioned too vertically in the coronal plane or too medial in the tibia lead to PCL impingement and abnormal tensile graft behavior when a transtibial tunnel technique is used. PCL impingement is the result of an error in coronal-plane positioning of the tibial tunnel and leads to loss of knee flexion and increased graft laxity and instability [26].

SURGERY
Patient Positioning
The patient is positioned supine on the operating table. After induction of anesthesia, an examination under anesthesia is performed. A tourniquet is placed around the proximal thigh of the operative leg. The operative leg is placed in a standard knee arthroscopy leg holder with the foot of the operating table flexed completely. Alternatively, the surgeon may decide to use a lateral post instead of a leg holder. The contralateral leg is positioned in a gynecologic leg holder with the hip flexed and abducted with mild external rotation (Fig. 1). Proper padding is used to ensure that no pressure is placed on the peroneal

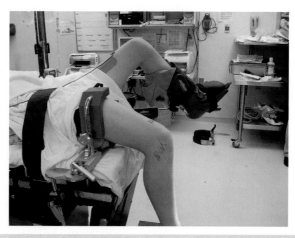

Fig. 1. Preferred patient set-up.

nerve and calf. Alternatively, surgeons can position the operative leg flexed over the side of the table using a lateral post and maintaining the contralateral leg extended on the operating table.

Preferred Surgical Technique

Tendon harvest

After sterile prep and drape, the leg is exsanguinated, and the tourniquet is inflated. A 2- to 3-cm incision is made along the anteromedial crest of the tibia centered three fingerbreadths below the medial joint line (Fig. 2). The incision should be positioned posterior enough on the anteromedial tibia so that the tip of the gloved finger reaches the popliteal crease medially (Fig. 3). A vertical incision allows the surgeon a more extensile incision should it be necessary to lengthen the incision for ease of hamstring harvest. Alternatively, oblique and horizontal incisions can be used. The incision is taken down sharply through the skin and subcutaneous fat to the sartorius fascia. The hamstring tendons are palpated, and the sartorius fascia is incised horizontal and parallel to the inferior border of the gracilis tendon. A finger is passed in the proximal direction deep to the sartorius fascia along the gracilis tendon. The finger is flexed to capture the gracilis tendon. A Penrose drain is looped around the tendon, and any fascial slips are released from the gracilis. The gracilis tendon is stripped from its musculotendinous junction using a blunt tendon stripper. The gracilis tendon is pulled, and the semitendinosus tendon is identified along the inferior border of the gracilis. An additional Penrose drain is looped around the semitendinosus tendon. Any fascial slips to the medial gastrocnemius originating from the inferior border of the semitendinosus tendon are identified and

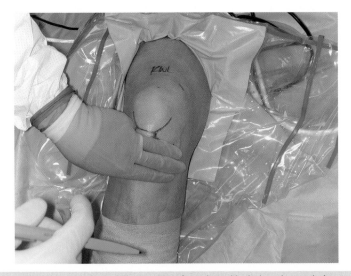

Fig. 2. Hamstring tendons generally are three fingerbreadths below the medial joint line.

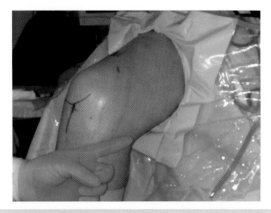

Fig. 3. Position the center of vertical or oblique harvest incisions so the gloved fingertip reaches the medial popliteal crease.

cut. The tendon then is stripped using an open-ended tendon stripper. The tendons are prepared by stripping the muscle from the tendon using scissors or a broad periosteal elevator. A stitch of the surgeon's choice is placed in the end of each tendon. The tendons are double-looped and sized using sizing sleeves (Fig. 4). The tendons should slide freely through the sizing sleeve. The tendons are removed subperiosteally from the anterior tibial crest at their common tendinous insertion including 5 to 10 mm of periosteum. A stitch of the surgeons' choice is placed in the common tendinous insertion. The tendons are stored in the sizing sleeve along with a damp sponge in a kidney basin on the back table. The kidney basin is covered with an occlusive plastic sheet to ensure the safety of the graft on the back table (Fig. 5).

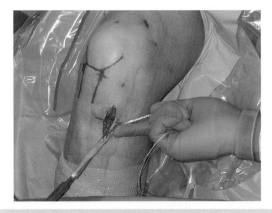

Fig. 4. Double-loop and size the tendons using sizing sleeves.

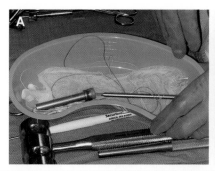
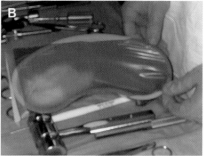

Fig. 5. (A) Prepared graft stored in appropriate sizing sleeve and saline-saturated sponge. (B) occlusive covering of graft stored on back table.

Portal placement

Inferolateral and inferomedial portals touching the edges of the patella tendon, starting 1 cm distal to the inferior pole of the patella, are established. Alternatively, a transpatellar inferolateral portal can be used with a medial portal placed along the medial border of the patella tendon. The medial portal must touch the edge of the patella tendon because, if it is placed more medially, the tibial guide may not stay seated in the intercondylar notch with the knee in full extension. An optional outflow portal can be established superiorly.

A diagnostic arthroscopy is performed. Meniscal or articular cartilage injuries are treated. The torn remnant ACL stump is identified and removed. It is not necessary to denude the tibial insertion of the native ACL tissue. In fact, retaining the insertion of the native ACL helps seal the edges of the ACL graft at the joint line and does not result in roof impingement if the tibial tunnel has been positioned appropriately. Synovium and soft tissue in the notch are removed to expose the lateral edge of the PCL (Fig. 6). Any of

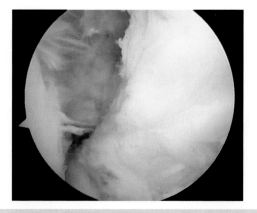

Fig. 6. Expose the superolateral leading edge of the posterior cruciate ligament.

the ACL origin from the over-the-top position is removed using an angled curette and shaver.

Tibial tunnel placement

The tibial guide is inserted through the medial portal. The guide is advanced into the intercondylar notch (**Fig. 7**). The tip of the guide is 9.5 mm wide. If the guide makes contact with and deforms the PCL as it enters the intercondylar notch, a lateral wallplasty is performed by removing bone in slivers 1 to 2 mm wide from the lateral wall until the tip of the guide passes into the notch without deforming the PCL. This technique creates an area wide enough for a graft 8 to 10 mm wide. No bone should be removed from the intercondylar roof, because the roof anatomy is crucial for proper positioning of the tibial guide pin in the sagittal plane using the 65° tibial guide. The lateral wallplasty fragments are removed.

The 65° tibial guide is inserted through the anteromedial portal that touches the medial edge of the patella tendon into the intercondylar notch between the PCL and lateral femoral condyle to ensure the notch is wide enough for the ACL graft (see **Fig. 7**). The knee then is extended fully (**Fig. 8**). The surgeon should determine arthroscopically that the tip of the guide is captured inside the notch and that the arm of the 65° tibial guide contacts the trochlea groove (**Fig. 9**). The patient's heel is placed on a Mayo stand to maintain the knee in maximum hyperextension. The surgeon stands on the lateral side of the leg and inserts the coronal alignment rod through the proximal hole in the guide. The 65° guide is rotated in varus and valgus until the coronal alignment rod is parallel to the joint and perpendicular to the long axis of the tibia. The combination bullet guide/hole changer is inserted into the 65° guide, and the bullet is advanced until it is seated against the anteromedial cortex of the tibia (**Fig. 10**). The guide then is lifted up while the knee is pushed into hyperextension and the coronal alignment rod parallel to the joint is maintained (see **Fig. 10**).

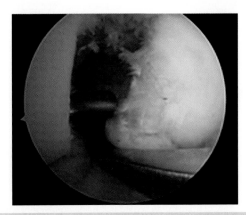

Fig. 7. The 65° guide positioned in the intercondylar notch.

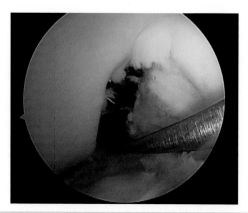

Fig. 8. Extend the knee while maintaining the tibial guide tip in the intercondylar notch.

The tibial guide pin is drilled through the lateral hole in the bullet until it strikes the guide intra-articularly. The bullet from the tibial guide is removed, and the guide is taken out of the notch. The guide pin is tapped into the notch and to assess its position (Fig. 11).

The tibial guide pin is positioned properly in the coronal plane when it enters the notch midway between the lateral edge of the PCL and the lateral femoral condyle. The guide pin should not touch the PCL (see Fig. 11). The tibial guide pin is positioned properly in the sagittal plane when there is 2 to 3 mm of space between the guide pin and the intercondylar roof with the knee in full extension. This space can be assessed by manipulating a nerve hook probe 2 mm wide between the between the guide pin and the intercondylar roof in the fully extended knee.

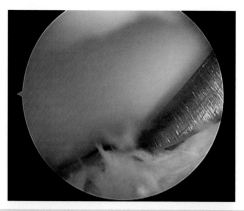

Fig. 9. Arthroscopic view of tibial guide seated in the intercondylar notch with the knee in full extension.

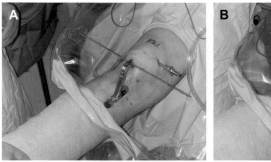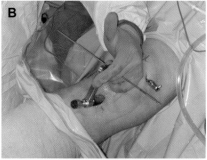

Fig. 10. (A) External view of 65° guide adjusted with the coronal alignment rod parallel to the knee joint. (B) External view of guide held in proper position by the surgeon during drilling of the tibial guide pin.

The tibial tunnel is prepared by reaming the tibial cortex with a reamer with the same diameter as the prepared ACL graft. A bone dowel is harvested from the tibial tunnel by inserting a bone dowel harvester and centering rod 8 mm in diameter over the tibial guide pin. A mallet is used to drive the bone dowel harvester until it reaches the subchondral bone. The dowel harvester containing the cancellous bone dowel is removed. If the tibial guide pin is removed with the bone dowel, it should be replaced by inserting it through an 8-mm reamer that has been reinserted into the tunnel created by the bone dowel harvester. The remainder of the tibial tunnel is reamed with the appropriate diameter reamer.

PCL impingement is checked by placing the knee in 90° of flexion and inserting the impingement rod into the notch. A triangular space at the apex of the

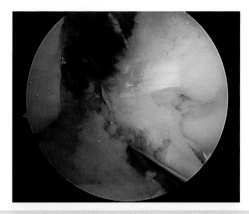

Fig. 11. Assess guide pin position. Note the entry of tibial guide pin below the remnant of ACL footprint tissue.

notch and no contact at the base of the notch between the PCL and impinge-ment rod confirms the absence of PCL impingement (**Fig. 12**). Roof impinge-ment is checked by placing the knee in full extension and inserting an impingement rod the same diameter as the tibial tunnel into the intercondylar notch (see **Fig. 12**). Free pistoning of the impingement rod in and out of the notch with the knee in full extension confirms the absence of roof impingement.

Femoral tunnel placement
The femoral tunnel is placed using the transtibial technique. The size-specific femoral aimer is inserted through the tibial tunnel with the knee in flexion. The size of the offset of the femoral aimer is based on the diameter of the ACL graft and is designed to create a femoral tunnel with a 1-mm back wall. The knee is extended, and the tip of the femoral aimer is hooked in the over-the-top position. The knee is allowed to flex, using gravity, until the femoral guide seats on the femur. The femoral aimer is rotated a quarter turn lateral away from the PCL, which positions the femoral guide pin farther down the lateral wall of the notch, minimizing PCL impingement. A pilot hole in the femur is drilled through the aimer, and both the guide pin and femoral aimer are removed (**Fig. 13**).

The femoral guide pin is redirected to shorten the femoral tunnel from 35 to 50 mm in length, using the following technique. The femoral guide pin is rein-serted into the pilot hole, and the knee is flexed to 90° to 100°. The guide pin is drilled through the lateral femoral cortex. A cannulated 1-inch reamer the same diameter as the ACL graft is passed over the guide pin. The femoral tunnel is reamed. The surgeon should confirm that the back wall of the femoral tunnel is only 1 mm thick (**Fig. 14**) and that the center of the femoral tunnel is midway between the apex and base of the lateral half of the notch. A femoral tunnel placed correctly down the sidewall does not allow room for a second

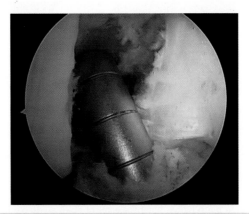

Fig. 12. The position of the impingement rod in the intercondylar notch.

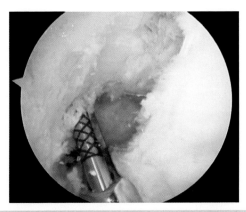

Fig. 13. The femoral aimer inserted through tibial tunnel with the femoral guide pin advanced into femur.

posterolateral tunnel. Finally, the length of the femoral tunnel should be measured using the transtibial tunnel depth gauge (**Fig. 15**).

Preparing the WasherLoc

The distal aspect of the tibial tunnel is exposed by removing a thumbnail portion of the surrounding soft tissue and periosteum. The counterbore aimer is inserted into the tibial tunnel. The guide is rotated to aim toward the fibular head. The counterbore awl is impacted to create a pilot hole in the tibial tunnel (**Fig. 16**). The anterior tibial tunnel is drilled using the counterbore reamer seated in the pilot hole and aimed toward the fibular head. The anterior distal tibial tunnel is reamed until flush with the posterior wall of the tibial tunnel (**Fig. 17**). The surgeon should not ream deeper than the posterior wall into the tibia. The bone from the flutes of the reamer is saved for bone grafting.

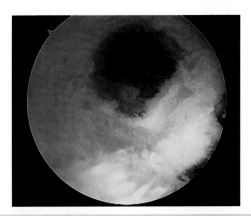

Fig. 14. Femoral tunnel position posterior with posterior wall 1 to 2 mm thick.

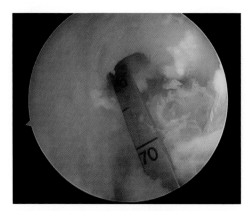

Fig. 15. Depth gauge showing femoral tunnel length.

EZLoc sizing and insertion

The EZLoc femoral fixation device is available in two diameters and three lengths to maximize fixation on the cortical bone and optimize bone tunnel surface area and graft length. For femoral tunnels of 7 or 8 mm in diameter, the 7/8 EZLoc device is used, and for femoral tunnels 9 or 10 mm in diameter, the 9/10 EZLoc device is used. For femoral tunnel lengths of 35 to 50 mm, as determined by depth gauge measurement, a "standard" length implant is chosen. For femoral tunnel lengths less than 35 mm, a "short" length implant is

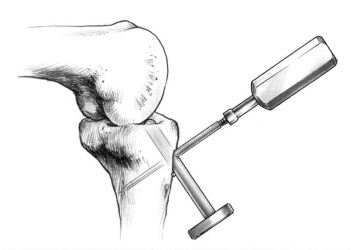

Fig. 16. Counterbore awl creates pilot hole in distal tibial tunnel aimed toward fibular head. (*From* Lawhorn KW, Howell SM. Scientific justification and technique for anterior cruciate ligament reconstruction using autogenous hamstring tendons and allogeneic soft tissue grafts. Orthop Clin North Am 2003;34(1):25.)

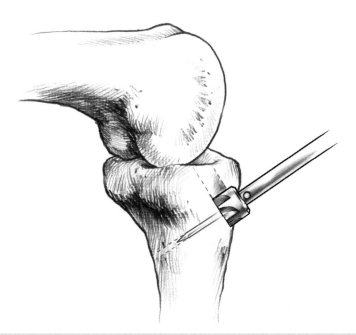

Fig. 17. Counterbore reamer removes distal anterior tibial tunnel until it is flush with posterior wall of tunnel and aimed toward fibular head. (*From* Lawhorn KW, Howell SM. Scientific justification and technique for anterior cruciate ligament reconstruction using autogenous hamstring tendons and allogeneic soft tissue grafts. Orthop Clin North Am 2003;34(1):26.)

used, and for femoral tunnel lengths greater than 50 mm, a "long" implant is used.

With the appropriate sized EZLoc device chosen, the passing pin connected to the EZLoc is inserted into the tibial tunnel and out of the femoral tunnel under arthroscopic visualization. The passing pin is pulled out the lateral thigh until the EZLoc implant is just outside the tibial incision and tibial tunnel entrance. The graft is passed through the loop of the EZLoc device. Alternatively, the graft can be passed through the device before the passing pin is inserted into the tibia and femoral tunnels. The ends of the graft are made even, and the sutures from the ends of the tendons are tied together. The distal aspect of the gold lever arm of the EZLoc is measured with a ruler, and a measurement corresponding to the length of the femoral tunnel is marked on the graft with a pen. This mark will ensure the EZLoc has passed lateral and proximal to the most proximal aspect of the femoral tunnel. The EZLoc is pulled into the joint and oriented so that the gold lever arm enters the femoral tunnel along the lateral wall of the tunnel (Fig. 18). Once the marked portion of the graft enters the femoral tunnel, the suture on the EZLoc and passing pin is cut. The passing pin is removed, and tension is pulled on the Ezloc suture, deploying the lever arm. The graft strands are tensioned, and the graft/EZLoc device is rocked

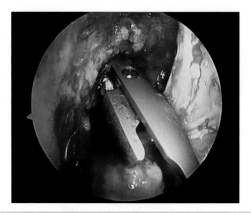

Fig. 18. EZLoc device with attached graft advanced into femoral tunnel with gold lever against lateral wall of tunnel.

back and forth to ensure the EZLoc is seated on the cortical bone of the lateral femur. The knee is cycled 20 to 30 times while tension on the graft is maintained.

WasherLoc tibial fixation
After cycling, the knee is positioned in full extension. All graft sutures are tied together, and an impingement rod is passed through the suture loops. The WasherLoc is assembled to the inserter and drill guide. The WasherLoc inserter awl is placed thorough the pilot hole, and the strands of the graft are captured within the long tines of the WasherLoc. An assistant puts tension

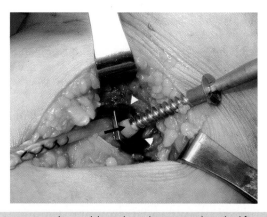

Fig. 19. WasherLoc screw advanced through washer to complete tibial fixation of graft. Bone wax (*black arrow*) is placed over the cutting threads of the self-tapping screw to protect the graft as the screw is inserted.

on all graft strands equally by pulling on the impingement rod. With all graft strands isolated between the long tines of the WasherLoc, the WasherLoc is driven into the graft and bone by a mallet. The inserter awl is removed, and a hole is drilled into the far cortex with a 3.2-mm drill through the drill guide. The drill guide is removed, and the length of the drill hole is determined. A small amount of bone wax is placed around the cutting threads of the appropriate-length self-tapping 6.0-mm cancellous screw. The screw is inserted through the WasherLoc, compressing the WasherLoc and graft against the posterior wall of the tibial tunnel (Fig. 19).

Bone graft tibial tunnel
The tibial tunnel dilator is inserted into the distal aspect of the tibial tunnel. In many cases the dilator can be advanced up the tunnel by hand. Alternatively, the dilator should be driven gently up the tibial tunnel by tapping lightly with a mallet. The plastic sleeve is placed over the tip of the bone dowel harvest tube and positioned so the plastic sleeve at the tip of the harvest tube is against the dilated opening of the tibial tunnel. The inner plunger rod is struck to deliver the cancellous bone dowel from the harvest tube into the tibial tunnel. The arthroscope is reinserted into the joint to inspect the graft. The knee is taken through a full range of motion to ensure there is no roof or PCL impingement (Fig. 20). The hamstring harvest site is closed in layers, the portal sites are closed, a sterile dressing is applied, and the tourniquet is deflated.

POSTOPERATIVE CARE AND REHABILITATION

Aggressive brace-free rehabilitation can be implemented safely with a DLHS graft using the EZLoc and WasherLoc fixation. Patients are allowed weight bearing as tolerated immediately after surgery. Patients can begin full active and passive range-of-motion exercises following surgery. The early focus is

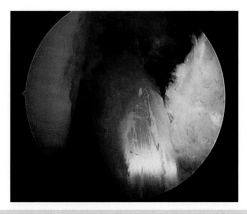

Fig. 20. Completed ACL reconstruction. Note the triangle formed at the high-noon position between the ACL graft and the superolateral fibers of the PCL.

on terminal extension and should be easy for the patient because the tibial tunnel is prepared with the knee in full extension. Once the patient has 110° of flexion, stationary bicycle exercises can begin. An exception is made for patients undergoing a concomitant meniscal repair. These patients are prescribed a brace and allowed partial weight bearing with the brace locked in full extension for 4 to 6 weeks. Range of motion is limited to zero to 90° for 4 to 6 weeks. Patients then progress to weight bearing as tolerated with unrestricted motion. Once full range of motion is achieved, patients can begin treadmill exercises and lower-extremity strengthening exercises. Jogging is typically begun at 10 to 12 weeks postoperatively. Agility exercises are begun after 12 weeks, and unrestricted full activity is allowed after 4 months if muscle strength is 85% of that of the contralateral normal knee. In patients undergoing a concomitant meniscal repair, unrestricted pivot activities are permitted after 6 months.

References

[1] Dopirak RM, Adamany DC, Steensen RN. A comparison of autogenous patellar tendon and hamstring tendon grafts for anterior cruciate ligament reconstruction. Orthopedics 2004;27(8):837–42 [quiz: 843–4].

[2] Gobbi A, Mahajan S, Zanazzo M, et al. Patellar tendon versus quadrupled bone-semitendinosus anterior cruciate ligament reconstruction: a prospective clinical investigation in athletes. Arthroscopy 2003;19(6):592–601.

[3] Sajovic M, Vengust V, Komadina R, et al. A prospective, randomized comparison of semitendinosus and gracilis tendon versus patellar tendon autografts for anterior cruciate ligament reconstruction: five-year follow-up. Am J Sports Med 2006;34(12):1933–40.

[4] Tow BP, Chang PC, Mitra AK, et al. Comparing 2-year outcomes of anterior cruciate ligament reconstruction using either patella-tendon or semitendinosus-tendon autografts: a non-randomised prospective study. J Orthop Surg (Hong Kong) 2005;13(2):139–46.

[5] Herrington L, Wrapson C, Matthews M, et al. Anterior cruciate ligament reconstruction, hamstring versus bone-patella tendon-bone grafts: a systematic literature review of outcome from surgery. Knee 2005;12(1):41–50.

[6] Laxdal G, Kartus J, Hansson L, et al. A prospective randomized comparison of bone-patellar tendon-bone and hamstring grafts for anterior cruciate ligament reconstruction. Arthroscopy 2005;21(1):34–42.

[7] Hamner DL, Brown CH Jr, Steiner ME, et al. Hamstring tendon grafts for reconstruction of the anterior cruciate ligament: biomechanical evaluation of the use of multiple strands and tensioning techniques. J Bone Joint Surg Am 1999;81(4):549–57.

[8] Noyes F. Biomechanical analysis of human ligament grafts used in knee-ligament repairs and reconstructions. J Bone Joint Surg Am 1984;66A:334–52.

[9] Yasuda K, Tsujino J, Ohkoshi Y, et al. Graft site morbidity with autogenous semitendinosus and gracilis tendons. Am J Sports Med 1995;23(6):706–14.

[10] Paulos LE, Wnorowski DC, Greenwald AE. Infrapatellar contracture syndrome. Diagnosis, treatment, and long-term followup. Am J Sports Med 1994;22(4):440–9.

[11] Kartus J, Movin T, Karlsson J. Donor-site morbidity and anterior knee problems after anterior cruciate ligament reconstruction using autografts. Arthroscopy 2001;17(9):971–80.

[12] Tomita F, Yasuda K, Mikami S, et al. Comparisons of intraosseous graft healing between the doubled flexor tendon graft and the bone-patellar tendon-bone graft in anterior cruciate ligament reconstruction. Arthroscopy 2001;17(5):461–76.

[13] Magen HE, Howell SM, Hull ML. Structural properties of six tibial fixation methods for anterior cruciate ligament soft tissue grafts. Am J Sports Med 1999;27(1):35–43.

[14] Brand J Jr, Weiler A, Caborn DN, et al. Graft fixation in cruciate ligament reconstruction. Am J Sports Med 2000;28(5):761–74.

[15] Singhatat W, Lawhorn KW, Howell SM, et al. How four weeks of implantation affect the strength and stiffness of a tendon graft in a bone tunnel: a study of two fixation devices in an extraarticular model in ovine. Am J Sports Med 2002;30(4):506–13.

[16] Greis PE, Burks RT, Bachus K, et al. The influence of tendon length and fit on the strength of a tendon-bone tunnel complex. A biomechanical and histologic study in the dog. Am J Sports Med 2001;29(4):493–7.

[17] Howell SM, Roos P, Hull ML. Compaction of a bone dowel in the tibial tunnel improves the fixation stiffness of a soft tissue anterior cruciate ligament graft: an in vitro study in calf tibia. Am J Sports Med 2005;33(5):719–25.

[18] Matsumoto A, Howell SM, Liu-Barba D. Time-related changes in the cross-sectional area of the tibial tunnel after compaction of an autograft bone dowel alongside a hamstring graft. Arthroscopy 2006;22(8):855–60.

[19] Howell SM, Hull ML. Aggressive rehabilitation using hamstring tendons: graft construct, tibial tunnel placement, fixation properties, and clinical outcome. Am J Knee Surg 1998;11(2):120–7.

[20] Chandratreya AP, Aldridge MJ. Top tips for RigidFix femoral fixation. Arthroscopy 2004;20(6):E59–61.

[21] Cuomo P, Edwards A, Giron F, et al. Validation of the 65 degrees Howell guide for anterior cruciate ligament reconstruction. Arthroscopy 2006;22(1):70–5.

[22] Howell SM, Lawhorn KW. Gravity reduces the tibia when using a tibial guide that targets the intercondylar roof. Am J Sports Med 2004;32(7):1702–10.

[23] Howell SM, Clark JA. Tibial tunnel placement in anterior cruciate ligament reconstructions and graft impingement. Clin Orthop Relat Res 1992;283:187–95.

[24] Howell SM. Principles for placing the tibial tunnel and avoiding roof impingement during reconstruction of a torn anterior cruciate ligament. Knee Surg Sports Traumatol Arthrosc 1998;6(Suppl 1):S49–55.

[25] Simmons R, Howell SM, Hull ML. Effect of the angle of the femoral and tibial tunnels in the coronal plane and incremental excision of the posterior cruciate ligament on tension of an anterior cruciate ligament graft: an in vitro study. J Bone Joint Surg Am 2003;85A(6):1018–29.

[26] Howell SM, Gittins ME, Gottlieb JE, et al. The relationship between the angle of the tibial tunnel in the coronal plane and loss of flexion and anterior laxity after anterior cruciate ligament reconstruction. Am J Sports Med 2001;29(5):567–74.

Clin Sports Med 26 (2007) 587–596

CLINICS IN SPORTS MEDICINE

ELSEVIER
SAUNDERS

Quadriceps Tendon—A Reliable Alternative for Reconstruction of the Anterior Cruciate Ligament

Joseph P. DeAngelis, MD[a,*], John P. Fulkerson, MD[a,b]

[a]Department of Orthopaedic Surgery, University of Connecticut School of Medicine, MARB 4th Floor, Farmington, CT 06032, USA
[b]Orthopedic Associates of Hartford, P.C., 499 Farmington Avenue, Suite 300 Farmington, CT 06032, USA

Reconstruction of the anterior cruciate ligament (ACL) has been shown to provide good results predictably [1–4]. In most cases, affected individuals can return to their desired sports with a stable knee. Most often, the ACL is reconstructed using the central portion of the patellar tendon or a double-looped semitendinosus/gracilis "hamstring" autograft [1,5–23]. Other potential sources of autologous tissue include the iliotibial band and the quadriceps tendon [24–31]. Increasingly, allograft tissue is being used as an alternative to decrease the morbidity associated with harvesting donor tissue [32–34]. Although these reconstruction techniques have well-documented clinical histories, each has specific drawbacks, inviting the development of a better ACL reconstruction graft alternative.

With correct surgical technique and no internal derangement of the knee, Kartus and colleagues [35] explained that problems related to the donor site can be grouped into general categories: (1) anterior knee pain and discomfort resulting from decreased function, including range of motion and muscular strength; (2) local discomfort caused by numbness, tenderness, or an inability to kneel; and (3) late tissue reaction at the donor site. Although anterior knee pain is the most commonly recognized complication of ACL reconstruction with patellar tendon, this technique also carries the additional risk of patella fracture and patellar tendon rupture. Harvesting the medial hamstring tendons for a looped semitendinosus/gracilis autograft can be complicated by injury to neighboring neurovascular structures, tendon amputation during the harvest, tendon rupture, and, in the long run, a decrease in terminal knee flexion strength. Although these complications are rare, their potential impact warrants

*Corresponding author. Department of Orthopaedic Surgery, University of Connecticut School of Medicine, MARB 4th Floor, Farmington, CT 06032. E-mail address: jpdeange lis@yahoo.com (J.P. DeAngelis).

0278-5919/07/$ – see front matter
doi:10.1016/j.csm.2007.06.005

concern and attention. Additionally, medial thigh hematoma and spasm pain are fairly common following hamstring harvest [36].

In an attempt to address these graft-specific issues, some surgeons have turned to the central quadriceps tendon. In 1984, Blauth [37] reported his technique for harvesting the central third of the quadriceps tendon with a block of patellar bone, which Stäubli [38] subsequently popularized in his series published in 1992.

The original description of this technique required harvesting a bone plug from the proximal pole of the patella to allow the same rigid fixation used in patellar tendon reconstructions. This method enjoyed some success, but removing a block of bone from the patella still carries the added risk of patella fracture.

In 1999, Fulkerson [39] revisited the technique hoping to decrease the morbidity of the graft harvest and the possibility of postoperative complications associated with the patellar bone plug. In this modified technique, the central third of the quadriceps tendon is harvested without bone to yield a robust free tendon autograft. Since 1996 Fulkerson has used the central quadriceps free tendon (CQFT) graft almost exclusively, including in high-level athletes, for both primary and revision ACL reconstruction.

When necessary, this free quadriceps tendon can be augmented with an EndoPearl (Linvatec, Largo, Florida), a polylactic acid ball, or a disk of bone to optimize fixation. Augmentation usually is not necessary, however. An Endo-Button (Smith & Nephew; Mansfield, Massachusetts) has been used for fixation on the femoral side.

Other authors have developed techniques using the central third of the quadriceps tendon as a soft tissue graft alone. Antonogiannakis and colleagues [40] described a method using absorbable cross pins (Rigid Fix; Mitek; Johnson & Johnson, Norwood, Massachusetts) to provide outlet fixation near the joint line in a free quadriceps tendon reconstruction. An alternative technique was developed by Kim and colleagues [41] and presented as the quadriceps tendon composite autograft. In this technique, a wafer of bone is harvested according to the original technique during preparation of the tibial tunnel and then is attached to the free end of the quadriceps tendon autograft. The addition of this bone plug to the tendinous portion of the graft is believed to augment distal fixation. With cancellous bone on each end of the graft, rigid fixation can be provided close to the anatomic origin and insertion of ACL to decrease the potential for creep and to increase the likelihood that the graft will heal into bone tunnels with the creation of Sharpey's fibers [42]. With Kim's technique, aperture fixation reduces the windshield-wiper effect, lessens concerns about graft abrasion, and helps address these concerns with all soft tissue reconstructions [43]. The authors' experience with Endo-Button fixation on the femoral side and quadriceps free tendon has not demonstrated a need for aperture fixation on the femoral side.

TECHNIQUE OF CENTRAL QUADRICEPS FREE TENDON ANTERIOR CRUCIATE LIGAMENT RECONSTRUCTION

The CQFT may be harvested through a short incision above the proximal patella extending proximally for 2 cm to 5 cm as needed. With experience harvesting the graft, and in most patients who are particularly concerned about cosmesis, the graft may be harvested well through a short incision.

Once the incision is made, the quadriceps tendon is exposed on its dorsal surface, and the vastus medialis is readily identified. The graft is best taken toward the medial-central aspect of the central quadriceps tendon, because this is its thickest part. One should start the incision for the tendon graft harvest at the proximal medial border of the vastus medialis using a #10 scalpel blade. The scalpel then is drawn from proximal to distal, establishing a graft 7 to 8 cm long measured from the proximal pole of the patella upwards (a #10 scalpel blade is just over 7 mm wide). An incision is made perpendicular to the dorsal surface of the quadriceps tendon to a depth of 6 to 7 mm (the quadriceps tendon is almost 10 mm thick at this point) [44]. After the medial border is established, a second incision is made parallel to the first incision, 9 to 10 mm lateral to the first incision and to a depth of 6 to 7 mm depth. Care is taken to avoid penetrating into the suprapatellar pouch, because leakage of fluid makes the harvest more difficult. With experience, it is uncommon to enter the pouch. Keeping the knee flexed to 90° helps the harvest by maintaining tension on the quadriceps. The surgeon should note that these incisions cut through both rectus femoris and intermedius portions of the quadriceps tendon, yielding a bilaminar graft that also is well suited to double-bundle ACL reconstruction if desired. There is a thin, fatty layer between the two, particularly at the more distal aspect. It is important to obtain portions of both components of the quadriceps tendon to obtain adequate depth. Ultimately, a tendon graft with a depth of 6 to 7 mm is desired. The depth of the patellar tendon averages about 4.9 mm [28].

Once the two initial incisions are made, a hemostat is used to define the posterior border of the tendon graft. The hemostat is spread generously at the posterior border of the desired graft size (Fig. 1) to define the distal insertion of the

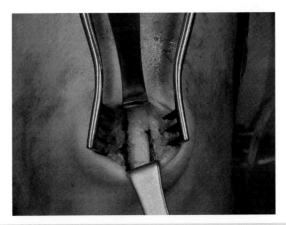

Fig. 1. A hemostat is used to define the posterior border of the tendon graft after the initial incisions are made, and the insertion of the quadriceps tendon at the patella is defined.

quadriceps tendon at the patella. The defined portion of the graft is incised and released distally, again spread with the hemostat. The tendon then is grasped with a uterine clamp (Fig. 2), and whipstitches are placed in the distal end of the tendon. The authors place two separate whipstitches with #5 nonabsorbable suture material or #2 Fiberwire (Arthrex; Naples, Florida). This procedure leaves four strands of #5 strength suture off the end of the tendon. According to Fulkerson and colleagues [45], only two whipstitches are needed on each side of the tendon to obtain optimal holding strength. At this point, the tendon is stripped proximally with Metzenbaum scissors, taking care to maintain selectively all fibers in the defined free tendon graft. This entire dissection takes place under direct visualization, taking care not to violate the graft or the adjacent quadriceps. Once the dissection has been completed to a level 7 to 8 cm above the patella, the free tendon graft is released proximally and taken to the back table. Nonabsorbable whip stitches are placed in both ends of the graft, again using the uterine clamp to hold it on a graft-preparation table.

The free tendon graft then may be placed into the tunnels that had been created for ACL reconstruction. Criteria for graft placement are the same as for any other free tendon graft. The free tendon should lie on the posterior border of the tibial tunnel so that this region is at the desired isometric location just posterior to the central aspect of the excised ACL. Tunnels are drilled to accommodate the graft. In most cases the tunnels range in size from 7 to 9 mm. Because the CQFT graft is bilaminar, including rectus and intermedius, it can be used easily for double-bundle ACL reconstruction.

The femoral tunnel should be drilled to a 35-mm depth, and when, as the authors prefer, an Endo-Button is used for fixation, an Endo-Button drill is used to penetrate the anterolateral cortex of the femur. The depth of the tunnel from the anterolateral cortex to the intra-articular opening of the femoral socket

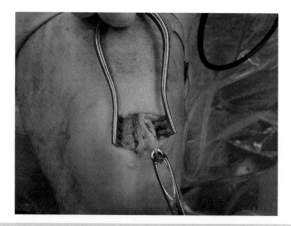

Fig. 2. Once released, the graft is held with a uterine clamp, and whipstitches are placed in the distal end.

is measured, and the graft is prepared with an Endo-Button, placing the sutures from one end of the free tendon graft through the central holes of the Endo-Button and then tying them immediately adjacent to the graft itself (Fig. 3). A #5 suture is used as a lead suture with a #2 suture in the other, trailing lateral hole of the Endo-Button. After the ACL graft sockets have been smoothed and prepared, the graft is drawn into the proper depth (the quadriceps tendon graft is marked at a point 2 to 2.5 cm from the end of the tendon graft to the point of fixation in the femoral notch end of the femoral socket), and the Endo-Button is deployed on femoral side. Because the sutures have been tied at the exact correct length, the graft will be seated securely in exactly the right position with 2 to 2.5 cm of quadriceps tendon graft in the femoral socket.

On the tibial side, the authors favor a bio-interference screw measuring 1 mm larger than the tunnel size. Nagarkatti and colleagues [46] have shown that this technique provides optimal fixation and, when combined with a button over the tibial tunnel, provides very secure fixation.

The graft harvest site at the proximal patella is explored for bleeding once the tourniquet is released. The trough where the tendon has been removed is left open, with only the peritenon closed over it. The skin is closed, and a compressive wrap is applied.

CLINICAL OUTCOMES OF ANTERIOR CRUCIATE LIGAMENT RECONSTRUCTION USING THE QUADRICEPS TENDON

Although not as widely studied as bone-tendon-bone or hamstring autografts, the current orthopedic literature provides considerable support for the quadriceps tendon autograft in ACL reconstruction. The original series published by Stäubli [47] helped generate enthusiasm for the technique published by Blauth [37] and established the quadriceps tendon as a desirable alternative for autologous soft tissue reconstructions.

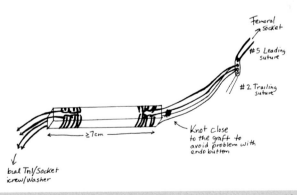

Fig. 3. After determining the length of the femoral tunnel, the graft is prepared for Endo-Button fixation. Sutures are placed from one end of the free tendon graft through the central holes of the Endo-Button and tied immediately adjacent to the graft itself.

Subsequent retrospective evaluations have supported further both the viability and longevity of the quadriceps tendon graft. The authors' recent long-term outcome study confirms that the CQFT is reliable for ACL reconstruction with good to excellent outcomes at more than 2 years of follow-up (unpublished data, DeAngelis and Fulkerson, 2007). This investigation demonstrated no donor-site morbidity and complete absence of anterior knee pain, proving that the CQFT is a reliable, pain-free, low-morbidity autograft alternative in ACL reconstruction.

In this single-surgeon series, all patients with more than 2 years follow-up after CQFT ACL reconstruction were asked to complete a subjective, objective, and functional evaluation of their reconstructed knee. Of 191 reconstructions, there were 5 graft failures (4%) and 1 infection requiring reoperation (0.5%). The average length of follow-up was 66 months (median, 67 months; range, 24–105 months) and the average International Knee Documentation Committee score at follow-up was 84.7 (median, 89.7; range, 14.9–100). No patient reported tenderness to palpation at the graft donor site, and knee range of motion was symmetric in all patients. Compared with the uninvolved knee, the average side-to-side difference in KT-1000 testing (as evaluated by an independent, unbiased physical therapist) was 1.2 mm at 20 pounds (median, 1.0; range, −2–6) and 1.8 mm at manual maximum testing (median, 1.2; range. 0.6–7.5). At manual maximum testing, 38 patients (86% of patients tested) had less than 3 mm side-to side difference. The single-leg hop test quotient was 0.96 (median, 0.95; range, 0.65–1.35). This study, together with Joseph's [48] data on short-term rehabilitation, suggests that the CQFT graft offers stability comparable to that of the other ACL graft reconstruction alternatives but with less short- and long-term morbidity, based on average follow-up of more than 5 years.

In 2004, Lee and colleagues [49] found that ACL reconstruction using a quadriceps tendon autograft showed satisfactory results with reduced donor-site morbidity. Sixty-seven ACL reconstructions were evaluated at a mean of 41 months (range, 27–49 months) and demonstrated a median laxity of 2 mm postoperatively. The Lysholm score improved postoperatively from 71 to 90 ($P < .05$). The peak extension torque of the quadriceps muscle was found to be 82% and 89% of that of the contralateral knee at 180°/second at 1 year and 2 years after surgery, respectively. Using congruence angle and Insall-Salvati ratio, the patellar position did not show any significant change after the graft was harvested. Only 4 of 41 patients (10%) complained of moderate pain on kneeling, and 1 patient complained of harvest-site tenderness. In this way, the quadriceps tendon harvested with bone is comparable to bone-patellar tendon-bone or hamstring tendon for ACL reconstruction.

Although the absence of anterior knee pain has been cited consistently as an advantage of the quadriceps tendon graft, the effect of the graft harvest on the extensor mechanism has been a concern despite comparable results in terms of knee stability and performance. In practice, extensor mechanics has not been a problem. In 2006, Joseph and colleagues [48] prospectively compared the early physical findings of hamstring, patellar tendon, and quadriceps tendon ACL reconstructions. They found that the quadriceps free tendon group achieved knee extension earlier than those reconstructed with patellar tendon and required less pain medication postoperatively than either hamstring or patellar tendon reconstruction patients. At testing to failure in cadaver knees, Adams and colleagues [50] established that the central quadriceps tendon is as strong after graft harvest as the patellar tendon is before a bone-tendon-bone harvest.

As additional support for this technique, Chen and colleagues [9] found satisfactory subjective and objective results at 4 to 7 years' follow-up using the quadriceps tendon-patellar bone autograft for ACL reconstruction. Of 38 patients treated, 32 patients (94%) achieved good or excellent results by Lysholm knee rating, and 26 patients (76%) had returned to moderate or strenuous activity at an average follow-up of 62 months (range, 48–84 months). In this study, the authors emphasized that the quadriceps tendon autograft has the advantage of being readily available.

When the quadriceps tendon is used for revision surgery, the results also have been highly acceptable. Garofalo and colleagues [51] retrospectively reviewed 31 patients in whom the central third of the quadriceps tendon was used for a revision ACL reconstruction using a two-incision technique. All patients demonstrated a positive pivot shift preoperatively, and 79% had radiographic evidence of tunnel malposition from the index surgery. At a minimum of 3 years' follow-up, 93% returned to sports, and no patient required an additional surgery following quadriceps tendon ACL revision. Five patients, however, had sensitive scars from the original surgery that affected their ability to kneel.

In a biomechanical comparison of the quadriceps tendon with bone plug and a traditional bone-patellar-tendon-bone construct, Dargel and colleagues [52] found comparable loading characteristics in the two grafts when tested to ultimate failure with a rising load angle using a 25-mm patellar bone plug. The study also illustrated the broad, deep insertion of the quadriceps tendon into the proximal patella.

Some have questioned the effect of harvesting the central third of the quadriceps tendon on the function of the extensor mechanism despite a lack of evidence supporting any difference between CQFT and bone-tendon-bone autografts [53]. Biomechanically, both Stäubli and colleagues [47] and Adams and colleagues [50] have demonstrated the relative strength of the quadriceps tendon autograft construct in comparison with the patellar tendon.

Stäubli and colleagues [47] compared a quadriceps tendon-patellar bone graft to a patellar tendon-patellar bone graft and found the patellar tendon to have a higher mean ultimate tensile stress and greater strain (elongation) on testing to failure. Correspondingly, Adams and colleagues [50] tested the residual quadriceps tendon after harvesting the central quadriceps free tendon as described by Fulkerson [39] and compared this tissue with the residual patellar tendon following a free patellar tendon harvest. They found both the native intact quadriceps tendon and the residual quadriceps tendon after harvest had a statistically higher strength at failure than the corresponding patellar tendon construct.

SUMMARY

The central quadriceps tendon provides a unique, low-morbidity ACL graft alternative. Both the quadriceps tendon-patellar bone graft and the free tendon graft are well supported in the literature as producing good to excellent outcomes at more than 2 years of follow-up. The decreased donor-site morbidity and absence of anterior knee pain suggest that the quadriceps free tendon autograft (without patellar bone) offers the clinician a reliable, pain-free, low-morbidity autograft alternative in ACL reconstruction. Recent short- and long-term data suggest that the CQFT may be the least morbid of all the currently used ACL autograft reconstruction alternatives.

References

[1] Bach BR Jr, Jones GT, Sweet FA, et al. Arthroscopy-assisted anterior cruciate ligament reconstruction using patellar tendon substitution. Two- to four-year follow-up results. Am J Sports Med 1994;22:758–67.

[2] Bach BR Jr, Jones GT, Hager CA, et al. Arthrometric results of arthroscopically assisted anterior cruciate ligament reconstruction using autograft patellar tendon substitution. Am J Sports Med 1995;23:179–85.

[3] Buss DD, Warren RF, Wickiewicz TL, et al. Arthroscopically assisted reconstruction of the anterior cruciate ligament with use of autogenous patellar-ligament grafts. Results after twenty-four to forty-two months. J Bone Joint Surg Am 1993;75:1346–55.

[4] Stapleton TR. Complications in anterior cruciate ligament reconstructions with patellar tendon grafts. Sports Medicine and Arthroscopy Review 1997;5:156–62.

[5] Aglietti P, Buzzi R, Menchetti PM, et al. Arthroscopically assisted semitendinosus and gracilis tendon graft in reconstruction for acute anterior cruciate ligament injuries in athletes. Am J Sports Med 1996;24:726–31.

[6] Alm A, Gillquist J. Reconstruction of the anterior cruciate ligament by using the medial third of the patellar ligament. Treatment and results. Acta Chir Scand 1974;140:289–96.

[7] Barber FA. Triple semitendinosus-cancellous bone anterior cruciate ligament reconstruction with Bioscrew fixation. Arthroscopy 1999;4:360–7.

[8] Brown CH Jr, Steiner ME, Carson EW. The use of hamstring tendons for anterior cruciate ligament reconstruction. Technique and results. Clin Sports Med 1993;12:723–56.

[9] Chen CH, Chuang TY, Wang KC, et al. Arthroscopic anterior cruciate ligament reconstruction with quadriceps tendon autograft: clinical outcome in 4–7 years. Knee Surg Sports Traumatol Arthrosc 2006;14:1077–85.

[10] Dandy DJ, Flanagan JP, Steenmeyer V. Arthroscopy and the management of the ruptured anterior cruciate ligament. Clin Orthop Relat Res 1982;167:43–9.

[11] Engstrom B, Wredmark T, Westblad P. Patellar tendon or Leeds-Keio graft in the surgical treatment of anterior cruciate ligament ruptures. Intermediate results. Clin Orthop Relat Res 1993;295:190–7.

[12] Graf B, Uhr F. Complications of intra-articular anterior cruciate reconstruction. Clin Sports Med 1988;7:835–48.

[13] Hamner DL, Brown CH Jr, Steiner ME, et al. Hamstring tendon grafts for reconstruction of the anterior cruciate ligament: biomechanical evaluation of the use of multiple strands and tensioning techniques. J Bone Joint Surg Am 1999;81:549–57.

[14] Jones KG. Reconstruction of the anterior cruciate ligament. J Bone Joint Surg Am 1963;45:925–32.

[15] Jones KG. Reconstruction of the anterior cruciate ligament using the central one-third of the patellar ligament. J Bone Joint Surg Am 1970;52:838–9.

[16] Kohn D, Sander-Beuermann A. Donor-site morbidity after harvest of a bone-tendon-bone patellar tendon autograft. Knee Surg Sports Traumatol Arthrosc 1994;2:219–23.

[17] Mohtadi NG, Webster-Bogaert S, Fowler PJ. Limitation of motion following anterior cruciate ligament reconstruction. A case-control study. Am J Sports Med 1991;19:620–5.

[18] Otero AL, Hutcheson L. A comparison of the doubled semitendinosus/gracilis and central third of the patellar tendon autografts in arthroscopic anterior cruciate ligament reconstruction. Arthroscopy 1993;9:143–8.

[19] Paulos LE, Rosenberg TD, Drawbert J, et al. Infrapatellar contracture syndrome. An unrecognized cause of knee stiffness with patella entrapment and patella infera. Am J Sports Med 1987;15:331–41.

[20] Puddu G. Method for reconstruction of the anterior cruciate ligament using the semitendinosus tendon. Am J Sports Med 1980;8:402–4.

[21] Sachs RA, Daniel DM, Stone ML, et al. Patellofemoral problems after anterior cruciate ligament reconstruction. Am J Sports Med 1989;17:760–5.

[22] Shelbourne KD, Trumper RV. Preventing anterior knee pain after anterior cruciate ligament reconstruction. Am J Sports Med 1997;25:41–7.

[23] Siegel MG, Barber-Westin SD. Arthroscopic-assisted outpatient anterior cruciate ligament reconstruction using the semitendinosus and gracilis tendons. Arthroscopy 1998;14:268–77.

[24] Bak K, Jörgensen U, Ekstrand J, et al. Results of reconstruction of acute ruptures of the anterior cruciate ligament with an iliotibial band autograft. Knee Surg Sports Traumatol Arthrosc 1999;7:111–7.

[25] Chen CH, Chuang TY, Wang KC, et al. Arthroscopic anterior cruciate ligament reconstruction with quadriceps tendon autograft: clinical outcome in 4–7 years. Knee Surg Sports Traumatol Arthrosc 2006;14(11):1077–85.

[26] Ekstrand J. Reconstruction of the anterior cruciate ligament in athletes, using a fascia lata graft: a review with preliminary results of a new concept. Int J Sports Med 1989;10:225–32.

[27] Eriksson E. Reconstruction of the anterior cruciate ligament. Orthop Clin North Am 1976;7:167–79.

[28] Fulkerson JP, Langeland R. An alternative cruciate reconstruction graft: the central quadriceps tendon. Arthroscopy 1995;11(2):252–4.

[29] Harris NL, Smith DAB, Lamoteaux L, et al. Central quadriceps tendon for anterior cruciate ligament reconstruction, part I: morphometric and biomechanical evaluation. Am J Sports Med 1997;25:23–8.

[30] Howe J, Johnson RJ, Kaplan MJ, et al. Anterior cruciate ligament reconstruction using quadriceps patellar tendon graft, part I: long-term follow-up. Am J Sports Med 1991;19:447–57.

[31] Nicholas JA, Minkoff J. Iliotibial band transfer through the intercondylar notch for combined anterior instability (ITPT procedure). Am J Sports Med 1978;6:341–53.

[32] Breitfuss H, Fröhlich R, Povacz P, et al. The tendon defect after anterior cruciate ligament reconstruction using the midthird patellar tendon—a problem for the patellofemoral joint? Knee Surg Sports Traumatol Arthrosc 1996;3:194–8.

[33] Jackson DW, Grood ES, Goldstein JD, et al. A comparison of patellar tendon autograft and allograft used for anterior cruciate ligament reconstruction in the goat model. Am J Sports Med 1993;21:176–85.

[34] Noyes FR, Barber-Westin SD. Reconstruction of the anterior cruciate ligament with human allograft. Comparison of early and later results. J Bone Joint Surg Am 1996;78:524–37.

[35] Kartus J, Stener S, Lindahl S, et al. Factors affecting donor-site morbidity after anterior cruciate ligament reconstruction using bone-patellar tendon-bone autografts. Knee Surg Sports Traumatol Arthrosc 1997;5:222–8.

[36] Carofino B, Fulkerson J. Medial hamstring tendon regeneration following harvest for anterior cruciate ligament reconstruction: fact, myth, and clinical implication. Arthroscopy 2005;21(10):1257–65.

[37] Blauth W. Die zweizügelige Ersatzplastik des vorderen Kreuzbandes aus der Quadricepssehne. Unfallheilkkunde 1984;87:45–51.

[38] Stäubli HU. The quadriceps tendon–patellar bone construct for ACL reconstruction. Sports Medicine and Arthroscopy Review 1997;5:59–67.

[39] Fulkerson J. Central quadriceps free tendon for anterior cruciate ligament reconstruction. Oper Tech Sports Med 1999;7(4):195–200.

[40] Antonogiannakis E, Yiannakopoulos CK, Hiotis I, et al. Arthroscopic anterior cruciate ligament reconstruction using quadriceps tendon autograft and bioabsorbable cross-pin fixation. Arthroscopy 2005;21(7):894, e1–5.

[41] Kim DW, Kim JO, You JD, et al. Arthroscopic anterior cruciate ligament reconstruction with quadriceps tendon composite autograft. Arthroscopy 2001;17(5):546–50.

[42] Rodeo SA, Arnoczky SP, Torzilli PA, et al. Tendon healing in a bone tunnel. J Bone Joint Surg Am 1993;75:1795–803.

[43] Ishibashi Y, Rudy TW, Livesay GA, et al. The effect of anterior cruciate ligament graft fixation site at the tibia on knee stability: evaluation using a robotic testing system. Arthroscopy 1997;13:177–82.

[44] Lairungruang W, Kuptniratsaikul S, Itiravivong P. The remaining patellar tendon strength after central one-third removal: a biomechanical study. J Med Assoc Thai 2003;86:1101–5.

[45] Fulkerson J, McKeon BP, Donahue BS, et al. The central quadriceps tendon as a versatile graft alternative in anterior cruciate ligament reconstruction: techniques and recent observations. Tech Orthop 1998;13(4):367–74.

[46] Nagarkatti DG, McKeon BP, Donahue BS, et al. Mechanical evaluation of a soft tissue interference screw in free tendon anterior cruciate ligament graft fixation. Am J Sports Med 2001;29(1):67–71.

[47] Staubli HU, Schatzmann L, Brunner P, et al. Mechanical tensile properties of the quadriceps tendon and patellar ligament in young adults. Am J Sports Med 1999;27(1):27–34.

[48] Joseph M, Fulkerson J, Nissen C, et al. Short-term recovery after anterior cruciate ligament reconstruction: a prospective comparison of three autografts. Orthopedics 2006;29(3): 243–8.

[49] Lee S, Seong SC, Jo H, et al. Outcome of anterior cruciate ligament reconstruction using quadriceps tendon autograft. Arthroscopy 2004;20(8):795–802.

[50] Adams DJ, Mazzocca AD, Fulkerson JP. Residual strength of the quadriceps versus patellar tendon after harvesting a central free tendon graft. Arthroscopy 2006;22(1):76–9.

[51] Garofalo R, Djahangiri A, Siegrist O. Revision anterior cruciate ligament reconstruction with quadriceps tendon-patellar bone autograft. Arthroscopy 2006;22(2):205–14.

[52] Dargel J, Schmidt-Wiethoff R, Schneider T, et al. Biomechanical testing of quadriceps tendon-patellar bone grafts: an alternative graft source for press-fit anterior cruciate ligament reconstruction? Arch Orthop Trauma Surg 2006;126(4):265–70.

[53] Pigozzi F, Di Salvo V, Parisi A, et al. Isokinetic evaluation of anterior cruciate ligament reconstruction: quadriceps tendon versus patellar tendon. J Sports Med Phys Fitness 2004;44(3): 288–93.

Clin Sports Med 26 (2007) 597–605

CLINICS IN SPORTS MEDICINE

ELSEVIER
SAUNDERS

Allograft Safety in Anterior Cruciate Ligament Reconstruction

Steven B. Cohen, MD[a,b,*], Jon K. Sekiya, MD[c]

[a]Rothman Institute Orthopaedics, 925 Chestnut Street, Philadelphia, PA 19107, USA
[b]Department of Orthopaedic Surgery, Thomas Jefferson University, 925 Chestnut Street,
Philadelphia, PA 19107, USA
[c]MedSport, Department of Orthopaedic Surgery, University of Michigan, 124 Frank Lloyd Wright
Drive, P.O. Box 0391, Ann Arbor, MI 48106, USA

Soft tissue allografts are an integral part of the surgical reconstruction of knee ligament, meniscus, and osteochondral injuries. Their increasing use in anterior cruciate ligament (ACL) reconstruction stems from an increased demand for a graft that allows decreased donor-site morbidity, decreased operative time, decreased postoperative pain, improved cosmesis, and earlier rehabilitation. A number of allografts currently are being used in ACL reconstruction, including bone-patella tendon-bone (BTB) (Fig. 1A and B), Achilles tendon, tibialis anterior or posterior tendon, hamstring tendons, and fascia lata (Fig. 2). The disadvantages associated with the use of allograft are the risk of disease or infection transmission, slower graft incorporation, cost, availability, and potential for immunologic response. In January, 2005 the American Orthopaedic Society for Sports Medicine organized a conference regarding allograft use and determined that although many studies have suggested that clinical outcomes of ligament reconstruction are equivalent for allograft and autograft tissue, these studies have methodologic flaws, and surgeons must be cautious regarding these results.

ALLOGRAFT USE IN THE UNITED STATES

The use of allografts in orthopaedic sports medicine has increased significantly during the last 15 years. The American Association of Tissue Banks (AATB) estimated by that in 2004 more than 1 million allografts were used by the 86 tissue banks that are members of the association [1]. An additional 64 tissue banks in the United States are not members of the AATB, so the total number of allografts used may have been more than 1.5 million. It has been estimated that nearly 300,000 ACL

*Corresponding author. Rothman Institute Orthopaedics, 925 Chestnut Street, Philadelphia,
PA 19105, USA. E-mail address: steven.cohen@rothmaninstitute.com (S.B. Cohen).

0278-5919/07/$ – see front matter
doi:10.1016/j.csm.2007.06.003
sportsmed.theclinics.com

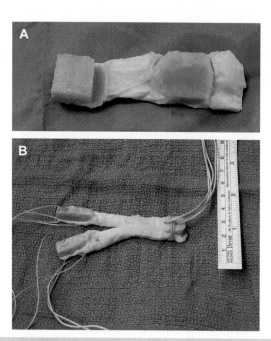

Fig. 1. Whole patellar tendon allograft. (*A*) To save costs and increase the number of avail-able grafts, tissue banks split patellar tendon allografts into two separate pieces. This is a whole graft that will be used because of its larger size and increased available collagen, which is another advantage of using allograft tissue. (*B*) A bifid-patellar tendon allograft that can be used for double-bundle ACL or posterior cruciate ligament reconstruction. This particular graft will be used for a double-bundle arthroscopic tibial inlay technique.

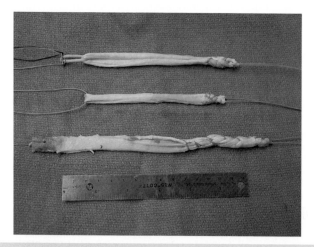

Fig. 2. Assorted allograft tissues: Semitendinosus tendon allograft (*top*), gracilis tendon allo-graft (*middle*), and Achilles tendon allograft (*bottom*).

reconstructions are performed each year in the United States, and approximately 20% (60,000) are performed using allograft [1].

INFECTION HISTORY

One of the greatest concerns regarding the use of allograft in ACL reconstruction is the transmission of bacterial or viral infection. Although *Morbidity and Mortality Weekly Report* (*MMWR*) published by the Centers for Disease Control and Prevention (CDC) provides information on infections after allograft use, there is no official reporting system. In the process of counseling to enable patients to give informed consent, potential recipients frequently ask about the risk of infection associated with implantation. Although specific sources have stated the risk of transmission of HIV and hepatitis to be approximately 1 in 1,600,000 [2], there are no recent or specific quoted rates, and the rates given "are based on extrapolations from incomplete and perhaps non-representative sources" [1].

There is important and useful information available regarding the rates of serum-positive viral infections in the general population. In a report by Strong and Katz [3] on living blood serum donors, the risk of transmission of HIV, hepatitis B, and hepatitis C were given as 1:400,000, 1:200,000, and 1:150,000, respectively. These figures, however, do not represent the number or the risk associated with soft tissue donors. As with blood donation, tissue banks perform standard tissue-recovery procedures that screen for high-risk behavior (eg, intravenous drug use) and test for infections (using cultures). Nonetheless, there have been a few, but widely known, reports of transmission of bacterial infection from musculoskeletal allografts.

The latest data released by the AATB from 2002 indicated only two reported bacterial infections from the 900,000 allografts distributed. (Reporting infections to the AATB is voluntary, however, and may not represent a true risk rate of 1 in 450,000 based on the 2002 data.) It also is possible that some infections occurring after allograft use were not attributed correctly to an infected allograft. Nearly 43% of all tissue banks are not members of or adhere to the standards of the AATB, which may increase the reported risk rate of bacterial infection.

In a study published by the CDC in 2004 in *The New England Journal of Medicine*, 70 cases of allograft-associated infection were reported [4]. There were six cases of hepatitis C infection and no cases of HIV infection since 1995. Fourteen patients were found to have Clostridium infections; all allografts were from the same tissue bank, which did not perform sterilization. More details from the CDC *MMWR* revealed one reported death occurring 4 days after femoral condyle (bone-cartilage) allograft implantation as a result of *C sordelli* infection [5]. Of the 26 reports of bacterial infections, 50% were infected with Clostridium species, and 11 patients were infected with gram-negative bacilli. Eighteen of the 26 infections occurred from allografts implanted for ACL reconstruction. Both these reports recommend that allograft safety be improved by maintaining validated processes for sterilization and culture to prevent allograft-associated infection. In addition, unless a sporicidal method is used, aseptically processed tissue should not be considered sterile and still represents a risk for Clostridium infection.

A recent study specifically aimed at positive cultures of implanted ACL reconstruction allografts from Spain found that 13.3% of the grafts were positive for culture 3 to 5 days after implantation [6]. None of the 24 patients had clinical knee infections, and all were treated with an antibiotic protocol. All patients were able to keep the reconstructed ACL allograft.

Although musculoskeletal allografts can improve quality of life significantly, infections associated with bacterial or viral contamination can result in serious morbidity and even death. The Food and Drug Administration (FDA) and CDC continue to regulate sterilization processes and investigate identified cases of allograft contamination in an effort to improve the efficacy and safety of allograft use.

GRAFT PROCUREMENT AND PREPARATION

Starting in May, 2005, all tissue banks in the United States were required to conform to the FDA's "Good Tissue Practice" guidelines, which mandate periodic inspections of tissue bank facilities and specify a minimum standard for tissue recovery, testing, and processing. Tissue banks are required to report adverse events to the FDA; individual surgeons and hospitals are encouraged to report specific reactions or complications, but this reporting is still voluntary. Before 1993, there were limited federal regulations overseeing the tissue bank industry; but regulation increased steadily, with the most recent formal guidelines set in 2005 [7].

The first stage for assuring safety in allograft use is the procurement phase. Tissue banks have established improved selection and testing protocols for donor tissue to ensure the absence of detectable infections, have improved production processes to remove or inactivate micro-organisms, and test tissue at appropriate stages of production to ensure freedom from detectable infections. Despite rigorous attempts to prevent bacterial or viral infection of donated tissue, there is no foolproof method of preventing this problem. One of the goals of donor screening is to prevent potential donations by individuals who are known to have a communicable disease (before or as a cause of death), who show signs of active infection, or who are at risk of infection as a result of high-risk behavior (eg, intravenous drug use or travel to regions with high infection rate). After a screening history, medical records review, and high-risk behavior review are performed, a physical examination is performed to detect physical evidence of high-risk behavior (eg, needle marks, signs of anal intercourse). Next, blood tests and tissue cultures are performed for infectious diseases including HIV (type I and II), hepatitis B, and hepatitis C. Some tissue banks have criteria for donor age and quality of tissue; however, the final determination to accept tissue is made by a "reasonable person" from the tissue bank (not required by the FDA to be a physician). Some tissue banks may accept known infectious tissue and count on sterilization to eliminate the risk of infection, but the AATB requires destruction of tissue if preprocessing cultures are positive for Clostridia or Group A Streptococcus.

Tissue retrieval is performed using standard operating room procedures. The tissue typically is rinsed with a surface bactericidal/antimicrobial disinfection solution without being formally sterilized. Each tissue bank has specific time restrictions on tissue retrieval. The tissue banking industry defines tissue sterility (the sterility assurance level) as a 1 in 1 million (1×10^{-6}) chance that a viable microbe is present in tissue that has undergone a sterilization process. To prevent the use of any conceivably contaminated allograft, the sterilization is validated by dunking ("spiking") the tissue in a solution with a known bioburden and subsequently measuring inactivation or removal of the organisms.

The two main processes for sterilization are irradiation and proprietary chemical processing (Table 1). Irradiation of soft tissue allografts is a delicate balancing act. Although irradiation up to 25 to 40 kGy can inactivate HIV and eliminate spores, the free radical formation resulting from these high doses has been shown to alter the biomechanics of the soft tissue graft significantly. Consequently, most tissue banks use low-dose irradiation ($\leq$ 4 kGy), which inactivates most micro-organisms but does not alter the effectiveness of the graft. Chemical sterilization entails a series of staged cleansing, disinfection, and rinsing in an effort remove lipids and cells to disinfect the tissue. The challenge in this technique is achieving enough penetration to sterilize the tissue. An additional sterilization technique, ethylene oxide gas, has excellent external sterilization properties but does not penetrate tissue penetration, and its by-products actually inhibit tissue remodeling. This technique was used more

Table 1
Proprietary tissue sterilization processes

Name	Wash type	Irradiation	Types of graft
Clearant Process (Clearant, Inc., Los Angeles, California)	Incubated in radioprotectant solution Dehydrated (freeze-dried)	50 kGy	Bone BTB
Allowash XG (LifeNet, Virginia Beach, Virginia)	Wet spin with H_2O_2 Proprietary solution soak Ultrasonification Antibiotic soak Dry spin Isopropyl alcohol soak	8.3 kGy	Bone BTB
Biocleanse (Regeneration Technologies, Inc., Alchua, Florida)	Proprietary soak Pressure fluctuations High vacuum Sterile water rinsle	25 kGy	Bone BTB
Tutoplast (Tutogen Medical, Inc., Alchua, Florida)	Acetone bath Osmotic bath: H_2O_2 washes Repeat acetone bath	20.1 kGy	Bone BTB

Abbreviation: BTB, bone-patellar tendon-bone.

than a decade ago, but it was found cause immune reactions and graft dissolution and currently is not recommended as a sterilization technique. Regardless of the sterilization technique used, poststerilized tissues should be cultured before implantation by the surgeon.

Tissues then are deep-frozen and stored at $-70°$ to $-80°C$ until surgery. Deep-freezing does not alter the biomechanics of the graft significantly; it does decrease antigenicity but does not destroy viruses such as HIV or hepatitis C virus. Ultimately it is the responsibility of the health care facility and surgeon to be aware of the techniques used by the tissue bank for harvesting and preparing grafts used in ACL surgery.

SAFETY
There are no definite data to help inform patients about the risks of transmission of HIV I/II, hepatitis B virus, or hepatitis C virus associated with the use of soft tissue allografts in orthopaedic surgery. It is prudent for the surgeon to be knowledgeable about the soft tissue bank's methods of preparation before using their allografts. Certainly the risks quoted in the literature for transmission of bacterial or viral infection from allografts are low, but those extremely rare instances of allograft infection have significant impact.

EFFICACY OF ALLOGRAFT IN ANTERIOR CRUCIATE LIGAMENT RECONSTRUCTION
Allograft use has become increasingly more common and has a number of advantages in ACL reconstruction. The most common allografts used are BTB, Achilles tendon, and hamstring or tibialis (anterior or posterior) tendons. The strength of nonirradiated allografts such as BTB or two-strand hamstring is equal to or greater than that of the native ACL [8], making allograft a good option for ACL reconstruction. Several animal studies in goats [9], dogs [10], and rabbits [11] have shown allografts are incorporated and remodeled as autografts are, although at a slower rate. Malinin and colleagues [12] conducted a human allograft retrieval study in nine patients who had undergone ACL reconstruction with allograft. The period between the reconstruction and the retrieval study ranged from 20 days to 10 years. This study found that remodeling of ACL grafts is a gradual or slow process, and complete remodeling and cellular replacement of the entire graft may require 3 years or longer. Additional animal studies have found that implantation of fresh tendon grafts with live donor cells display an inflammatory and rejection response [13]. These living cells in fresh allografts have a short survival time and quickly are replaced by host cells; this finding suggests that allografts that do not contain viable donor cells may avoid the immunologic response and potentially may incorporate more rapidly [14].

Despite the basic science differences between allografts and autografts, clinical studies have not found significant differences between the grafts when used for ACL reconstruction. A number of studies have shown comparable good-to-excellent results for either graft [15–18], but several other studies suggest there is greater laxity in knees with ACL reconstruction with allograft than with autograft [19–21]. The overall consensus is that allografts are comparable to autografts in restoring stability, range of motion, and subjective knee scores. In addition, allografts are useful for revision ACL reconstruction when autograft was used for the primary reconstruction. A number of studies have shown that allograft use in the revision setting is efficacious in improving symptoms, stability, functional limitation, and subjective knee scores [20,22–24].

INDICATIONS FOR USE

In 2007, the indications for the use of allografts in ACL reconstruction are not concrete. Many sports medicine physicians who perform ACL reconstructions prefer to use one type of graft for consistency and reproducibility. Some prefer allograft for its decreased morbidity and shorter operative times; others prefer autograft to avoid discussions with patients about disease transmission. It is difficult, however, to perform multiligament surgery around the knee without the using allograft or the contralateral knee autograft because of the number of grafts required for that reconstruction.

The authors prefer to approach graft selection for ACL reconstruction on an individual basis. They allow the patient to make an informed decision about the graft type used for the ACL reconstruction. They use the following general guidelines to counsel their patients:

> For patients who are less active, require sooner return to work, and desire less pain, the authors prefer to use allograft soft tissue, either tibialis tendon, or BTB allograft.
> For patients who are sprinters/hurdlers or elite-level athletes who require full terminal flexion strength or earlier return to sports, they prefer to use BTB autograft.
> For patients who have a history of patellar-femoral pain or who are high-level athletes without a history of hamstring problems, they prefer to use the quadrupled semitendinosus/gracilis autograft.
> For any patient who wants to avoid the risks of infection associated with allografts, they use strictly autograft tissue.
> They usually do not use Achilles tendon allograft, quadriceps tendon autograft, or contralateral knee grafts for ACL reconstructions.

SUMMARY

Allograft tissue seems to provide an excellent option for reconstruction of the ACL in the primary and revision setting. Certainly there are risks and benefits for the use of each graft available for ACL reconstruction. The advantages of using allograft are decreased donor-site morbidity, decreased operative time, decreased postoperative pain, improved cosmesis, and earlier rehabilitation. The disadvantages are the risks of disease or infection transmission, slower graft incorporation, cost, availability, and potential for immunologic response. Although in general the risks of using allograft tissue in ACL reconstruction are low, the consequences of complications associated with disease or infection transmission or of recurrent instability secondary to graft failure are large. Surgeons should provide patients with the information available regarding allograft risks and should have thorough knowledge of the source and preparation of the grafts by their tissue bank before implantation for ACL reconstruction.

References

[1] The American Orthopaedic Society for Sports Medicine Conference on Allografts in Orthopaedic Sports Medicine. Keystone (CO), July 14–17, 2005.

[2] Stevenson S, Arnoczky SP. Transplantation of musculoskeletal tissues. In: Simon SR, editor. Orthopaedic basic science: biology and biomechanics of the musculoskeletal system. Rosemont (IL): American Academy of Orthopaedic Surgeons; 2000. p. 567–79.

[3] Strong DM, Katz L. Blood-bank testing for infectious diseases: how safe is blood transfusion? Trends Mol Med 2002;8:355–8.

[4] Kainer MA, Linden JV, Whaley DN, et al. Clostridium infections associated with musculoskeletal-tissue allografts. N Engl J Med 2004;350:2564–71.

[5] Centers for Disease Control and Prevention. Update: allograft-associated infections—United States 2002. Morb Mortal Wkly Rep 2002;51:207–10.

[6] Diaz-de-Rada P, Barriga A, Barroso JL, et al. Positive culture in allograft ACL-reconstruction: what to do? Knee Surg Sports Traumatol Arthrosc 2003;11:219–22.

[7] Joyce MJ. Safety and FDA regulations for musculoskeletal allografts: perspectives of an orthopaedic surgeon. Clin Orthop 2005;435:22–30.

[8] Noyes FR, Butler DL, Grood ES, et al. Biomechanical analysis of human ligament grafts used in knee ligament repairs and reconstructions. J Bone Joint Surg 1984;66A:344–52.

[9] Jackson DW, Grood ES, Goldstein JD, et al. A comparison of patellar tendon autograft and allograft used for anterior cruciate ligament reconstruction in the goat model. Am J Sports Med 1993;21:176–85.

[10] Nikolaou P, Seaber A, Glisson R, et al. Anterior cruciate ligament allograft transplantation: long term function, histology, revascularization, and operative technique. Am J Sports Med 1986;14:348–60.

[11] Sabiston P, Frank C, Lam T, et al. Allograft ligament transplantation. a morphological and biochemical evaluation of a medial collateral ligament complex in a rabbit model. Am J Sports Med 1990;18:160–8.

[12] Malinin TI, Levitt RL, Bashore C, et al. A study of retrieved allografts used to replace anterior cruciate ligaments. Arthroscopy 2002;18:163–70.

[13] Arnoczky SP, Warren RF, Ashlock MA. Replacement of the anterior cruciate ligament using a patellar tendon allograft: an experimental study. J Bone Joint Surg 1986;68A:376–85.

[14] Tom JA, Rodeo SA. Soft tissue allografts for knee reconstruction in sports medicine. Clin Orthop 2002;402:135–56.

[15] Harner CD, Olson E, Irrgang JJ, et al. Allograft versus autograft anterior cruciate ligament reconstruction: 3- to 5-year outcome. Clin Orthop 1996;324:134–44.

[16] Peterson RK, Shelton WR, Bomboy AL. Allograft versus autograft patellar tendon anterior cruciate ligament reconstruction: a 5-year follow-up. Arthroscopy 2001;17:9–13.

[17] Poehling GG, Curl WW, Lee CA, et al. Analysis of outcomes of anterior cruciate ligament repair with 5-year follow-up: allograft versus autograft. Arthroscopy 2005;21:774–85.

[18] Shelton WR, Papendick L, Dukes AD. Autograft versus allograft anterior cruciate ligament reconstruction. Arthroscopy 1997;13:446–9.

[19] Barrett G, Stokes D, White M. Anterior cruciate ligament reconstruction in patients older than 40 years: allograft versus autograft patellar tendon. Am J Sports Med 2005;33:1505–12.

[20] Grossman MG, ElAttrache NS, Shields CL, et al. Revision anterior cruciate ligament reconstruction: three- to nine-year follow-up. Arthroscopy 2005;21:418–23.

[21] Uribe JW, Hechtman KS, Zvijac JE, et al. Revision anterior cruciate ligament surgery: experience from Miami. Clin Orthop 1996;325:91–9.

[22] Fagelman M, Freedman KB. Revision reconstruction of the anterior cruciate ligament: evaluation and management. Am J Orthopsychiatry 2005;34:319–28.

[23] Fox JA, Pierce M, Bojchuk J, et al. Revision anterior cruciate ligament reconstruction with nonirradiated fresh-frozen patellar tendon allograft. Arthroscopy 2004;20:787–94.

[24] Noyes FR, Barber-Westin SD, Roberts CS. Use of allografts after failed treatment of rupture of the anterior cruciate ligament. J Bone Joint Surg 1994;76A:1019–31.

Fresh-Frozen Allograft Anterior Cruciate Ligament Reconstruction

Matthew L. Busam, MD[a],
John-Paul H. Rue, MD, LCDR, MC, USN[b],
Bernard R. Bach, Jr, MD[c],*

[a]Cincinnati Sports Medicine Research and Education Foundation, Cincinnati, OH, USA
[b]Department of Orthopaedics, National Naval Medical Center, Bethesda, MD, USA
[c]Division of Sports Medicine, Rush University Medical Center, 1725 West Harrison St. Suite 1063, Chicago, IL 60612, USA

Reconstruction of the anterior cruciate ligament (ACL) with allograft tissue has emerged as an excellent option for a variety of patients. This article reviews the indications for allograft ACL reconstruction, graft options, and technique for allograft use.

INDICATIONS FOR ANTERIOR CRUCIATE LIGAMENT RECONSTRUCTION

For most active patients, reconstruction of the ACL provides an excellent chance of functional recovery and is preferred to activity modification and bracing. The literature is replete with numerous series of successful reconstructions using a variety of graft choices [1–16]. The decision to proceed with reconstruction should be made only after determining the patient's occupation, activity level, and expectations. Sedentary patients and those willing to attempt activity modification can consider nonoperative treatment [17]. No specific chronologic age is a contraindication [18,19]. Longitudinal studies traditionally have demonstrated that active patients have not been able to return to unrestricted function with an ACL-deficient knee [20–23]. The authors' indications for surgical reconstruction of the ACL-injured knee are outlined in Box 1.

GRAFT CHOICE

Once the decision has been made to proceed with reconstruction, graft choice becomes the next important factor to consider. At Rush University Medical Center, bone-patellar tendon-bone (BTB) autograft has been the primary graft choice for more than 20 years. The percentage of patients receiving allograft

Research performed at Rush University Medical Center, Chicago, Illinois.

*Corresponding author. E-mail address: brbachmd@comcast.net (B.R. Bach, Jr).

> **Box 1: Indications for ACL reconstruction**
>
> Active lifestyle, sport, and/or occupation
>
> Participation in hard-cutting, decelerating sports for more than 5 hours/week
>
> Associated repairable meniscus tear
>
> Recurrent instability
>
> High skill level
>
> Social considerations
>
> Multi-ligament knee injury
>
> KT-1000 (MEDmetric Corporation, San Diego, California) side-to-side differences of more than 3 mm
>
> Failed conservative treatment with bracing

reconstruction has increased from 2% our between 1986 and 1996 to almost 50% in 2006 [4]. The option of using allograft typically is discussed with patients who are more than 40 years of age, have evidence of degenerative joint disease or patellofemoral pain, or have insufficient or poor-quality donor tissue for autograft [4]. Patients who have multi-ligament knee injuries those who hope for an accelerated rehabilitation are others for whom the use of allograft tissue is an option (Box 2) Although available data indicate excellent clinical results in the population of older (age > 30 years) patients undergoing allograft reconstruction [4,10,24–26], this information cannot be extrapolated to patients aged 16 to 25 years involved in collision sports. Because long-term data on allograft use in this population are lacking, the authors do not routinely recommend allograft use for these patients.

TISSUE BANKING AND ALLOGRAFT PREPARATION

Fresh-frozen allograft tissue is the most common preparation technique [27]. In this process, the tissue is harvested under sterile conditions, cultured, and then is frozen while serologic tests are performed. After soaking in antibiotic solution, it is packaged and can be frozen for up to 5 years [28]. Cells do not survive this

> **Box 2: Considerations for allograft reconstruction**
>
> Age greater than 40 years
>
> Radiographic evidence of mild degenerative joint disease
>
> Moderate patellofemoral crepitation or pain symptoms
>
> Petite stature
>
> Donor graft tissue of questionable quality
>
> Request for allograft tissue
>
> Multi-ligament injuries
>
> Need for accelerated rehabilitation

process [28]. Freeze-dried allografts also are commonly used. Also known as "lyophilization," this process begins with sterile harvest of the tissue, which is frozen while serologic tests are performed and then is soaked in antibiotic solution. The tissue is refrozen and lyophilized to reduce the moisture content to less than 5%. It is packaged and stored for up to 5 years [28]. It must be rehydrated before use [29].

The possibility of disease transmission is an issue paramount to the patient and the surgeon. Significant numbers of musculoskeletal allografts are used in a variety of procedures each year (650,000 in 1999) [30]. The American Association of Tissue Banks [31] and the Food and Drug Administration have set guidelines for tissue harvest and processing; however, multiple case reports from the Centers for Disease Control and Prevention have demonstrated possible disease transmission [30,32]. HIV transmission has been reported as well [33]. Secondary sterilization with irradiation conceivably could eliminate viral vectors. A dose of 3 megarads (30,000 Gy) of gamma irradiation is necessary to sterilize fresh-frozen allograft [34], but this dose causes significant mechanical and material deficiencies in allograft tissue [35]. Therefore, irradiation at this dose as an effort to sterilize the graft terminally is not recommended [36]. Lower-dose irradiation is used commonly to sterilize tissue without compromising biomechanical function [27]. Despite the federal guidelines for allograft tissue banking and harvesting, the harvest, processing, and storage of allograft tissue continues to evolve [37]. The surgeon must be aware of the tissue bank used at his or her institution and be sure that appropriate precautions are taken during harvest and preservation to ensure that contaminated or mechanically compromised tissues are not used [38]. Allograft safety issues are discussed further elsewhere performed in this issue.

ALLOGRAFT CHOICE

The authors' preferred allograft tissue is a fresh-frozen BTB graft. They use this graft for several reasons. Fresh-frozen tissue does not require rehydration and has been well studied, clinically [39] and from a basic science standpoint [40]. It allows use of identical instrumentation for autograft or allograft procedures. It also allows bone-to-bone healing and rigid interference fixation. In addition, the authors have had success with its use in both primary and revision situations [4,41]. Other allograft options include a hemipatellar tendon, quadriceps tendon, Achilles tendon, or soft tissue graft, such as hamstring or tibialis tendons. Each of these choices has potential benefits and potential shortcomings. Graft–construct mismatch can be a significant problem with the use of BTB grafts, especially if a graft from a tall donor is used for a shorter patient. This difference can be magnified if a hemipatellar tendon is used. A hemipatellar tendon is a longitudinally bisected whole patellar tendon, allowing one extensor mechanism to provide two useable grafts. This technique results in a tendon that has a functionally longer soft tissue component than a central-third graft. When a hemipatellar allograft, is used, the discrepancy in length must be accounted for: the surgeon should order a graft that is several millimeters shorter than typically ordered for a whole tendon, because the functional soft tissue length will be longer once is it prepared. It is advisable to inform the bone bank of the patient's height and provide length parameters to reduce the likelihood of a significant graft–construct mismatch.

Some tissue banks are not able to provide whole BTB or even hemipatellar tendon grafts readily, and lower-volume surgeons may be unable to obtain them on a consistent basis. In this case, becoming comfortable with the preparation and fixation techniques for alternative graft choices is recommended.

The use of Achilles tendon allografts is a common and accepted alternative to BTB allograft [25,42–44]. With its ample distal bone stock and long, broad tendinous portion, the Achilles tendon allograft offers the combined advantages of bony fixation and the versatility for graft sizing and alternative soft tissue fixation methods. In a cost-comparison study, Cole and colleagues [45] found that the average cost of an ACL reconstruction procedure using Achilles tendon allograft was less than that for a BTB autograft ACL reconstruction procedure, despite a cost of more than $400 for the Achilles tendon allograft. The authors cited several reasons for the cost difference, including decreased operating room time and fewer inpatient admissions.

Ample bone is available at the distal calcaneal attachment of the Achilles tendon allograft to construct a bone block of varying sizes. The broad proximal tendon allows larger graft sizes if needed. These two variables make the Achilles tendon allograft an ideal graft choice, particularly for revision ACL reconstruction. Early clinical results by Levitt and colleagues [44] reported up to 87% satisfactory results using Achilles tendon allografts. More recently, Poehling and colleagues [25] validated these results, demonstrating similar long-term successful results with their primary ACL reconstructions using either BTB autograft or Achilles tendon allograft (Fig. 1).

BONE-PATELLAR TENDON-BONE ALLOGRAFT SURGICAL TECHNIQUE

A single preoperative dose of antibiotics is administered before surgical "timeout" and patient positioning. At this point, the surgeon should confirm the

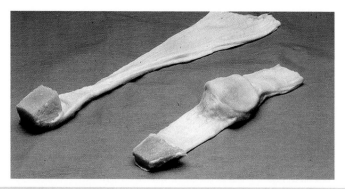

Fig. 1. Unprepared Achilles tendon (*top*) and whole bone-patellar tendon-bone (*bottom*) allografts.

availability of the appropriate allograft tissue. After anesthesia is initiated, an examination of the affected and unaffected knees is performed. The Lachman test, anterior and posterior drawer, pivot-shift testing, varus/valgus stress, and posterolateral instability at 30° and 90° should be performed and graded. It is crucial that other ligamentous pathology be diagnosed, because unrecognized path laxities can contribute to ACL reconstruction failure [46,47]. One must be cautious of ACL pseudolaxity in the event of posterior cruciate ligament deficiency. Once a positive pivot-shift test confirms ACL deficiency, the allograft can be thawed for preparation. The graft should not be placed directly into the warm saline solution, because it can become edematous and hypertrophy. It is best thawed by keeping the plastic covering on the tendon while it is in the solution. Alternatively, thawing the graft can begin once diagnostic arthroscopy confirms the ACL deficiency.

Diagnostic Arthroscopy

The inferolateral viewing portal is established just adjacent to the patellar tendon. This more medially based location allows improved visualization of the over-the-top position. Thorough evaluation of the suprapatellar pouch, medial and lateral gutters, and medial, lateral, and posterior compartments then is performed. Meniscal pathology, chondral injuries, and loose bodies are noted and addressed.

Allograft Preparation

The thawed allograft is inspected to confirm tissue integrity. Its soft tissue length is measured and recorded. The central third of the tendon is harvested similarly to autograft harvest (Fig. 2). A trapezoidal patellar plug 25 mm in length and 10 mm wide is harvested along with a triangular tibial plug of the same dimensions. To avoid splintering, care should be taken to avoid forcible levering of the bone plugs from their beds.

The bone blocks are trimmed with a small rongeur to remove sharp edges and ensure that they fit through a 10-mm sizing tube. The femoral plug should have a slight bullet contour to facilitate easy graft passage. When the plugs are adequately shaped, two holes are drilled through the cancellous portion of the

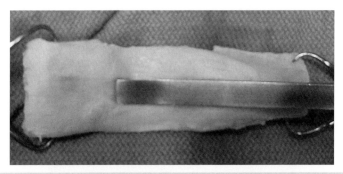

Fig. 2. An osteotome marks the central third of an unprepared bone-patellar tendon-bone allograft.

tibial bone plug parallel to the cortical surface using a 0.062-in Kirschner wire (K-wire). A No. 5 Ticron suture (Tyco; Waltham, Massachusetts) is placed in each hole. Placing the suture holes parallel to the cortex reduces the likelihood of lacerating the sutures as the interference screw is placed during graft fixation. If a pull-through method of graft passage is used, drill holes and sutures should be placed through the cortex of the femoral bone plug to reduce the possibility of the sutures cutting through the plug during graft passage [48]. Finally, the cancellous side of the tendo-osseous interface of the femoral plug and the cortical edge of the tibial plug are defined with a sterile marking pen for later assessment of graft orientation in the tunnels (Fig. 3). After preparation, the graft should be wrapped in a moist sponge and placed in a kidney basin on the main instrument table. All operative personnel should be informed of the graft's location to ensure its safety.

Tibial Tunnel and Notch Preparation

For an allograft technique, the only incision necessary, other than the arthroscopic portals, is a 1.5- to 2-cm incision placed 2 to 3 cm inferior and 2 to 3 cm medial to the tibial tubercle. A medially based periosteal window is created in the tibial metaphysis through this incision to allow tibial tunnel placement. Débridement of the intercondylar notch should be carried back to the over-the-top position for proper assessment of this landmark. The goal of the notchplasty is an opening of 10 mm between the lateral wall of the intercondylar notch and the lateral edge of the posterior cruciate ligament to prevent impingement of the graft in the notch. The notchplasty is completed from anterior to posterior using a bur to expand the notch superiorly and laterally to prevent graft impingement in full extension. The final configuration should resemble a smooth, rounded Roman arch rather than a pointed Gothic arch (Fig. 4). This configuration allows easier placement of the aiming guide at the 10:30 or 2:30 positions (depending on the side of the body); with a more steeply oriented arch configuration, the offset aimer can have a tendency to slide proximally (ie, toward the 11:30 or 12:30 position). A probe then is used to feel for appropriate placement

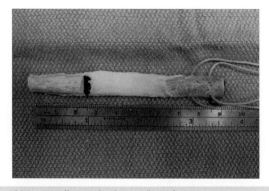

Fig. 3. A prepared bone-patellar tendon-bone allograft.

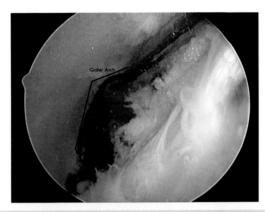

Fig. 4. Arthroscopic photograph demonstrating the preferred smooth Roman arch configuration for notchplasty, as opposed to the pointed Gothic arch (*solid black line*).

at the over-the-top position. On the tibial side, the ACL stump should be debrided fully to reduce the potential development of a Cyclops lesion [49–52].

Once the notch has been prepared adequately, a tibial drill guide is used to position the intra-articular position of the guide pin. The guide is set based on the "n + 10 rule," by adding 10 to the tendinous graft length to set the guide in degrees (eg, 45 mm + 10 = 55 degrees). This calculation, a modification of the "n + 7 rule" advocated by Miller [53,54], assists in matching the graft and tunnel lengths. Generally, the tibial guide is set at a 55° angle and occasionally is increased to 60° for longer tendons. Accurate pin placement can be directed by three parameters: (1) the posterior aspect of the tibial ACL footprint; (2) 5 mm lateral to the medial tibial spine; and (3) 7 mm anterior to the posterior cruciate ligament [55–57]. A simple general reference point is 3 to 4 mm posterior to the posterior edge of the anterior horn of the lateral meniscus. The guide is placed through a small accessory inferomedial transpatellar tendon stab wound made with the aiming stylet placed where the tibial tunnel will enter the joint (Fig. 5) This modification allows excellent mobility of the aiming device and easy medial-to-lateral orientation of the aimer. Because the orientation of the tibial tunnel affects the placement of the femoral tunnel, this technique ensures that the femoral tunnel entrance is low enough on the lateral wall to control rotational as well as anterior-posterior translation. The tunnel should be in the midline of the notch in the coronal plane; the goal is to place the subsequent femoral tunnel at the 10:30 position on a right knee and at 1:30 on a left knee.

When the stylet is positioned properly on the plateau, the sleeve of the guide is pushed to the cortical surface where the tibial tunnel will begin and is oriented to allow proper alignment in the coronal plane. The guide pin then is drilled just past the tibial plateau. The leg is extended to confirm proper placement, preventing graft impingement in the superior notch in full extension.

The guide pin then is tapped into the roof of the intercondylar notch to stabilize the pin. It is overdrilled with a cannulated reamer 1 mm larger than the

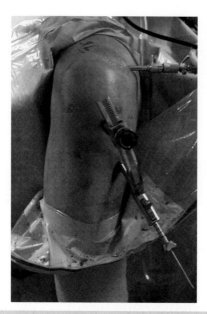

Fig. 5. The tibial aiming stylet placed through a transpatellar tendon stab incision. Note how the aimer can be positioned easily to allow proper orientation of the tunnel to provide correct placement of the femoral tunnel.

tibial bone block (typically 10 or 11 mm). The tunnel is plugged with a rubber stopper, and a shaver is used to remove osteochondral fragments from the intra-articular opening of the tibial tunnel. A chamfer reamer and a curved hand rasp are used successively to smooth the posterior edge of the tunnel's proximal opening. These measures help ensure that the femoral guide wire is not placed too far anteriorly, provide a smooth posterior surface against which the graft will lie, and reduce the likelihood of having to extend the knee to position the femoral offset aimer in the over-the-top position.

Femoral Tunnel

The two primary goals in drilling the femoral tunnel are to avoid blowout of the posterior cortical wall and to avoid creating a vertical femoral tunnel. With these objectives in mind, a femoral offset guide is inserted through the tibial tunnel, passed through the joint, and hooked at the over-the-top position. The guide then is positioned and rotated to achieve proper orientation (ie, 10:30 on a right knee (Fig. 6) and 1:30 on a left knee). If a 10-mm femoral tunnel is to be drilled, a 7-mm offset guide will leave a 2-mm shell of posterior cortical bone and reduce the likelihood of a blowout. When the guide is anchored properly, the guide pin is drilled to a depth of about 3.5 cm. To ensure the integrity of the posterior cortical wall, a tunnel footprint is reamed 10 mm into the femur before the tunnel is fully reamed (Fig. 7). The footprint is probed to confirm cortical stability and an appropriate thickness of 1 to 2 mm. The

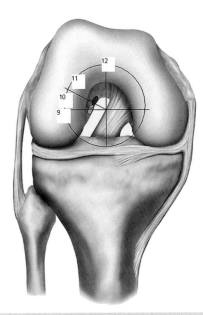

Fig. 6. Superimposed clock face demonstrates appropriate femoral tunnel placement.

tunnel then is reamed to a depth of 35 mm, which allows some flexibility if graft recession is needed to address a construct mismatch. The integrity of the femoral tunnel should be confirmed once again by inserting the arthroscope retrograde through the tibial tunnel and examining the femoral socket.

Graft Passage and Fixation

When the tibial and femoral tunnels are established, the graft is retrieved from the back table. A push-in technique is used for graft passage: a two-pronged

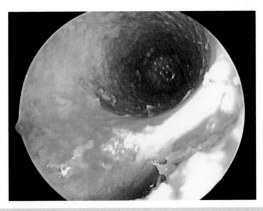

Fig. 7. Arthroscopic photograph of the femoral footprint. The intact cortical rim confirms that no blowout has occurred.

pusher is placed at the femoral tendo-osseous junction and used to push the graft retrograde through the tibial tunnel. The femoral bone plug is inserted with the cortex oriented posteriorly and in the coronal plane. A curved hemostat is placed through the inferomedial portal to grasp the femoral bone plug as it enters the joint. It should be grasped at the proximal–middle third junction of the bone plug to facilitate guiding the graft into the femoral socket. The soft tissues around the tibial tunnel entrance are retracted so that the tibial bone plug seats easily within the tibial tunnel.

Alternatively, based on preference, a pull-through technique can be used. When this method is used, the graft must be prepared with drill holes and passing sutures in the femoral bone plug as well as in the tibial bone plug. These passing sutures are passed through the eye of a Beath pin, and the Beath pin is pulled up through the tibial tunnel, across the joint, and through the femoral tunnel and femur; it exits the skin of the anterolateral thigh. The knee must be hyperflexed when the Beath pin is drilled to ensure that it exits the thigh distal to the drapes and tourniquet, to avoid contamination. The femoral passing sutures are pulled tight as the graft is brought into the joint, and a probe is used to help orient the cortical surface of the plug posteriorly.

Before the femoral bone plug is fully seated in its tunnel, a flexible 14-in guide pin is placed on the anterior aspect of the bone plug through the inferomedial portal. If the femoral bone plug is slightly intra-articular at this point, it acts as a skid for the guide wire. The leg should be flexed to approximately 110°, and the guide pin should slide effortlessly into the tunnel adjacent to the bone plug graft interface. Flexion allows the pin and screw to be placed parallel to the femoral bone plug. To ensure that the screw remains on the anterior aspect of the bone plug, a small indentation can be made with an arthroscopic curette or hemostat at the superior lateral outlet of the tunnel [58]. The femoral bone plug then is seated flush against the articular surface using a satellite pusher (Fig. 8). If the plug protrudes slightly from the distal tibial tunnel, the femoral bone plug can be recessed in its tunnel using the satellite pusher. When the graft is suitably positioned, a 7 × 25 mm metal interference screw is advanced halfway into the femoral tunnel (Fig. 9). One must be sure that the screw is not twisting graft fibers, risking laceration. The screw should be placed parallel to the bone plug because screw divergence of more than 15° can compromise fixation [59–61]. Once proper placement is confirmed, the guide pin is removed before the screw is seated fully. The quality of fixation is tested by cycling the knee several times with tension on the tibial sutures. The graft then is examined in full extension to ensure there is no notch impingement. In full extension, 3 to 5 mm of clearance between the graft and the roof of the notch is preferred. In the event of impingement, the notchplasty can be revised to improve clearance [62].

Before tibial fixation, the graft is rotated 180° toward the lateral wall of the intercondylar notch to shorten the graft and orient the cortical surface of the bone plug anteriorly. The leg is brought out to full extension, and firm tension is applied to the tibial sutures. The guide wire is placed along the anterior

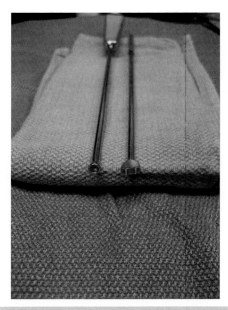

Fig. 8. The satellite (*left*) and two-pronged (*right*) pushers used during the push-in technique.

aspect of the tibial bone plug, and a 9 × 20 mm metal interference screw is used to secure the graft. The interference screw is placed anteriorly on the cortical plug surface. Cancellous-to-cancellous fixation is biomechanically superior to cortical-to-cancellous fixation [63]. Anterior placement has less divergence associated with screw placement. The graft then is viewed with the arthroscope to assess the orientation and tension (Fig. 10). Lachman and pivot-shift tests are performed to confirm the integrity of the reconstruction.

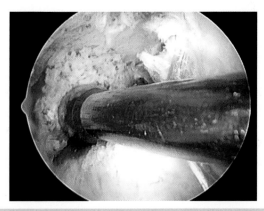

Fig. 9. Arthroscopic photograph of the metal interference screw advancing into the femoral tunnel.

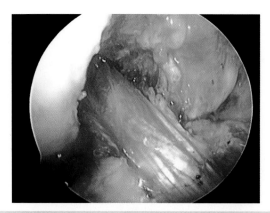

Fig. 10. Arthroscopic photograph of final graft orientation and placement.

Graft–Construct Mismatch

In the case of graft tunnel mismatch there are several options for salvage. Although recessing the femoral tunnel is one option, doing so increases the likelihood of lacerating the graft as the screw encounters the soft tissue component. In marked construct mismatches, one could use femoral suspension fixation (EndoButton; Smith and Nephew Endoscopy; Andover, Massachusetts) to recess the graft further while avoiding the risk of graft laceration with an interference screw. Another option is rotating the graft up to 540°. This procedure shortens the graft by approximately 5 to 6 mm, or 10% of its initial length [64]. Recent biomechanical data suggest that this rotation might place increased strain on the graft during cyclic loading [65], but the significance of this increased strain is unknown, because adverse clinical outcomes have not been reported [66].

For more significant mismatch, a free tibial bone block technique can be performed. In this technique, the tendon is resected sharply from the bone plug, and a Krackow suture is placed in the tendon. After the femoral side of the graft is secured, the bone plug is placed anterior to the soft tissue within the tibial tunnel while tension is maintained on the graft and the bone plug to prevent dislodgement. Interference screws are placed along the cortical edge of the plug [67]. Clinical results with this technique have been consistent with those of standard fixation [68].

ACHILLES TENDON ALLOGRAFT TECHNIQUE

Bone Block Preparation

Typically, a 25 × 10 mm bone block is fashioned from the distal bony calcaneal attachment of the graft. If needed, a larger bone block may be constructed, particularly in revision settings. Similar to BTB allograft preparation, the bone block is contoured and sized to slide easily through the appropriate sizing tube. Two holes are drilled through the cancellous portion of the bone plug parallel to the cortical surface using a 0.062-in K-wire. A #5 nonabsorbable braided suture is placed in each hole if a pull-through technique is to be used.

Soft Tissue Preparation

The preparation of the tendinous portion of the graft is similar to the preparation of other soft tissue grafts. The tendon is tabularized and may be contoured, depending on the desired size of the graft. Depending on the tibial fixation method chosen, the tendon graft length can be determined after passing the graft and securing the femoral fixation. This procedure has the advantage of eliminating mismatch of graft length. Charlick and Caborn [69] have described an alternative method of preparing soft tissue grafts that involves tightly grouped compression sutures in an attempt to form a tight bundle of collagen and suture. This technique allows interdigitation of the interference screw with the sutures and graft, enhancing screw capture.

Fixation

Numerous methods are available for both femoral and tibial fixation, including interference screws, staples, spiked washers, or other commercially available fixation devices. Commonly, the bone block is placed in the femur, and a metal interference screw is used, similar to the technique described for BTB graft fixation [5]. Tibial fixation may be performed by a variety of methods, with either staples or a spiked washer-and-screw construct. The initial pullout strength of each of these devices has been described in detail by several authors [5,67,70,71] and is beyond the scope of this article. Zamorano and Gold [72] described a novel technique for reversing the Achilles allograft, placing the bone plug distally on the tibia and using an EndoButton CL (Smith and Nephew; Andover, Massachusetts) for femoral fixation. Their technique is useful in revision ACL reconstruction procedures with significant bone loss and tibial tunnel widening, because it allow secure bone-to-bone fixation and bone blocks of varying sizes as needed.

REHABILITATION

ACL reconstruction has been performed on an outpatient basis at Rush University Medical Center since 1993. Intraoperatively, a motorized cooling pad and a drop-lock knee brace are applied. Patients receive a 30-tablet supply of oral narcotic pain medication. An aggressive rehabilitation course begins on the day of surgery with a session on crutch walking and a review of heel slides, prone heel hangs, quadriceps and hamstring sets, patellar mobilizations, and straight leg raises to be done in the first week. The authors believe that continuous passive motion machines are not indicated for routine ACL reconstruction and eliminated these machinesfrom their rehabilitation protocol in 1993. The authors' reoperation rate has been 1% to 2% for symptomatic knee flexion contractures since transitioning to outpatient ACL surgery. This rate is lower than that observed when patients used a continuous passive motion machine for either 1 or 3 days postoperatively (1986–1993). Every patient is seen on postoperative day one for a dressing change to reduce the likelihood of

SteriStrip (3M, St. Paul, Minnesota) blistering and to assess the need for aspiration of any hemarthrosis. Sutures and SteriStrips are removed 8 to 12 days postoperatively. Between 2 and 4 weeks postoperatively, the patient begins toe raises, closed chain extension exercises, hamstring curls, and stationary bicycling, in addition to weight-bearing stretching of the gastrocnemius and soleus. The drop-lock knee brace is locked in extension for ambulation until the patient demonstrates normal quadriceps control. In allograft patients this control often is seen by 10 days. Patients can remove the brace for closed-chain strengthening activities. By 8 to 12 weeks postoperatively, patients who have normal range of motion can advance to straight-ahead running and closed-chain strengthening. Patients can return gradually to participation in high-level athletics between 4 and 6 months, postoperatively.

SUMMARY

Reconstruction of the ACL provides consistently good to excellent results allowing return to work and sport. Allograft tissue is an alternative to autografts when appropriate donor tissue is not available or advisable for other reasons. The technique and results for allograft use are similar to those for autograft, making its use appropriate in a variety of clinical scenarios.

References

[1] Aglietti P, Buzzi R, D'Andria S, et al. Arthroscopic anterior cruciate ligament reconstruction with patellar tendon. Arthroscopy 1992;8:510–6.

[2] Aglietti P, Buzzi R, Giron F, et al. Arthroscopic-assisted anterior cruciate ligament reconstruction with central third patellar tendon. Knee Surg Sports Tramatol Arthrosc 1997;5: 138–44.

[3] Bach BR Jr. Patellar tendon autograft for ACL reconstruction. In: Miller MD, Cole BJ, editors. Textbook of arthroscopy. Philadelphia: Elsevier; 2004. p. 645–56.

[4] Bach BR Jr, Aadalen KJ, Dennis MG. Primary anterior cruciate ligament reconstruction using fresh-frozen, nonirradiated patellar tendon allograft: minimum 2-year follow-up. Am J Sports Med 2005;33:284–92.

[5] Bach BR Jr, Jones GT, Sweet FA, et al. Arthroscopy-assisted anterior cruciate ligament reconstruction using patellar tendon substitution. Am J Sports Med 1994;22:758–67.

[6] Bach BR Jr, Levy ME, Bojchuk J, et al. Single-incision endoscopic anterior cruciate ligament reconstruction using patellar tendon autograft minimum two-year follow up evaluation. Am J Sports Med 1998;36:30–40.

[7] Bach BR Jr, Tradonsky S, Bojchuk J, et al. Arthroscopically assisted anterior cruciate ligament reconstruction using patellar tendon autograft. Five- to nine-year follow-up evaluation. Am J Sports Med 1998;26:20–9.

[8] Buss DD, Warren RF, Wickiewicz TL, et al. Arthroscopically assisted reconstruction of the anterior cruciate ligament with use of autogenous patellar-ligament grafts. Results after twenty-four to fourty-two months. J Bone Joint Surg Am 1993;75:1346–55.

[9] Deehan DJ, Salmon LJ, Webb VJ, et al. Endoscopic reconstruction of the anterior cruciate ligament with an ipsilateral patellar tendon autograft. A prospective longitudinal five-year study. J Bone Joint Surg Br 2000;82:984–91.

[10] Indelli PF, Dillingham MF, Fanton GS, et al. Anterior cruciate ligament reconstruction using cryopreserved allografts. Clin Orthop Relat Res 2004;420:268–75.

[11] Johma NM, Pinczewski LA, Clingeleffer AJ, et al. Arthroscopic reconstruction of the anterior cruciate ligament with patellar-tendon autograft and interference screw fixation. The results at seven years. J Bone Joint Surg Br 1999;81:775–9.

[12] Nedoff DD, Bach BR Jr. Arthroscopic anterior cruciate ligament reconstruction using patellar tendon autografts: a comprehensive review of contemporary literature. Am J Knee Surg 2001;14:243–58.

[13] Otto DD, Pinczewski LA, Clingeleffer AJ, et al. Five-year results of single-incision arthroscopic anterior cruciate ligament reconstruction with patellar tendon autograft. Am J Sports Med 1998;26:181–8.

[14] Podskubka A, Kasal T, Vaculik J, et al. [Arthroscopic reconstruction of the anterior cruciate ligament using the transtibial technique and a graft from the patellar ligament: results after 5-6 years]. Acta Chir Orthop Traumatol Cech 2002;69:169–74 [in Czech].

[15] Shelbourne KD, Gray T. Anterior cruciate ligament reconstruction with autogenous patellar tendon graft followed by accelerated rehabilitation. A two- to nine- year followup. Am J Sports Med 1997;25:786–95.

[16] Spindler KP, Kuhn JE, Freedman KB, et al. Anterior cruciate ligament reconstruction autograft choice: bone-tendon-bone versus hamstring does it really matter? A systematic review. Am J Sports Med 2004;32:1986–95.

[17] Ciccotti MG, Lombardo SJ, Nonweiler B, et al. Non-operative treatment of ruptures of the anterior cruciate ligament in middle aged patients. J Bone Joint Surg Am 1994;76: 1315–21.

[18] Novak PJ, Bach BR Jr, Hager CA. Clinical and functional outcome of anterior cruciate ligament reconstruction in the recreational athlete over the age of 35. Am J Knee Surg 1996;9: 111–6.

[19] Plancher KD, Steadman JR, Briggs KK, et al. Reconstruction of the anterior cruciate ligament in patients who are at least forty years old. A long-term follow-up and outcome study. J Bone Joint Surg Am 1998;80:184–97.

[20] Barrack RL, Bruckner JD, Kneisl J, et al. The outcome of non-operatively treated complete tears of the anterior cruciate ligament in active young adults. Clin Orthop Relat Res 1990;259:192–9.

[21] Daniel DM, Stone ML, Dobson BE, et al. Fate of the ACL-injured patient. A prospective outcome study. Am J Sports Med 1994;22:632–44.

[22] Hawkins RJ, Misamore GW, Merritt TR. Followup of the acute nonoperated isolated anterior cruciate ligament tear. Am J Sports Med 1986;14:205–10.

[23] Noyes FR, Mooar PA, Matthews DS, et al. The symptomatic anterior cruciate deficient knee. Part I, the long term functional disability in athletically active individuals. J Bone Joint Surg Am 1983;65:154–62.

[24] Kuechle DK, Pearson SE, Beach WR, et al. Allograft anterior cruciate ligament reconstruction in patients over 40 years of age. Arthroscopy 2002;18:845–53.

[25] Poehling GG, Curl WW, Lee CA, et al. Analysis of outcomes of anterior cruciate ligament repair with 5-year follow-up: allograft versus autograft. Arthroscopy 2005;21(7): 774–85.

[26] Peterson RK, Shelton WR, Bomboy AL. Allograft versus autograft patellar tendon anterior cruciate ligament reconstruction: a 5-year follow-up. Arthroscopy 2001;17:9–13.

[27] Barbour SA, King W. The safe and effective use of allograft tissue. In: Scott WN, editor. 4th edition, Insall and Scott surgery of the knee, vol. 1. Philadelphia: Elsevier; 2006. p. 686–92.

[28] Shelton WR, Treacy SH, Dukes AD, et al. Use of allografts in knee reconstruction: I. Basic science aspects and current status. J Am Acad Orthop Surg 1998;6(3):165–8.

[29] Bechtold JE, Eastlund DT, Butts MK, et al. The effects of freeze-drying and ethylene oxide sterilization on the mechanical properties of human patellar tendon. Am J Sports Med 1994;22:562–6.

[30] Centers for Disease Control and Prevention. Update: allograft-associated bacterial infections—United States, 2002. Morb Mortal Wkly Rep 2002;51:201–10.

[31] American Association of Tissue Banks. AAOS and AATB information for patients. McLean (VA): American Association of Tissue Banks; 2003.

[32] Centers for Disease Control and Prevention. Septic arthritis following anterior cruciate ligament reconstruction using tendon allografts–Florida and Louisiana, 2000. Morb Mortal Wkly Rep 2001;50:1081–3.

[33] Asselmeier MA, Caspari RB, Bottenfield RB. A review of allograft processing and sterilization techniques and their role in transmission of the human immunodeficiency virus. Am J Sports Med 1993;21:170–5.

[34] Fideler BM, Vangsness CT Jr, Moore T, et al. Effects gamma irradiation on the human immunodeficiency virus. A study in frozen human bone-patellar ligament-bone grafts obtained from infected cadavera. J Bone Joint Surg Am 1994;76:1032–5.

[35] Gibbons MJ, Butler DL, Grood ES, et al. Effects of gamma irradiation on the initial mechanical and material properties of goat bone-patellar tendon-bone allografts. J Orthop Res 1988;6:95–102.

[36] Schwartz HE, Matava ML, Proch FS, et al. The effect of gamma irradiation on anterior cruciate ligament allograft biomechanical and biochemical properties in the caprine model at time zero and at 6 months after surgery. Am J Sports Med 2006;34:1747–55.

[37] Vangsness CT Jr. Soft-tissue allograft processing controversies. J Knee Surg 2006;19:215–9.

[38] American Academy of Orthopaedic Surgeons. Advisory statement #1011: use of musculoskeletal tissue allografts [position statement]. J Am Acad Orthop Surg 2001.

[39] Indelicato PA, Bittar ES, Prevot TJ, et al. Clinical comparison of freeze-dried and fresh frozen patellar tendon allografts for anterior cruciate ligament reconstruction of the knee. Am J Sports Med 1990;18:335–42.

[40] Nikolaou PK, Seaber AV, Glisson RR, et al. Anterior cruciate ligament allograft transplantation. Long-term function, histology, revascularization, and operative technique. Am J Sports Med 1986;14(5):348–60.

[41] Fox JA, Pierce M, Bojchuk J, et al. Revision anterior cruciate ligament reconstruction with nonirradiated fresh-frozen patellar tendon allograft. Arthroscopy 2004;20:787–94.

[42] Jackson DW, Kurzweil PR. Allografts in knee ligament surgery. In: Scott WN, editor. Ligament and extensor mechanism injuries of the knee. St Louis (MO): Mosby; 1991. p. 349–60.

[43] Noyes FR, Barber-Westin SD. Reconstruction of the anterior cruciate ligament with human allograft. Comparison of early and later results. J Bone Joint Surg Am 1996;78(4):524–37.

[44] Levitt RL, Malinin TI, Posada A, et al. Reconstruction of anterior cruciate ligaments with bone-patellar tendon-bone and Achilles tendon allografts. Clin Orthop Relat Res 1994;303:67–78.

[45] Cole DW, Ginn TA, Chen GJ, et al. Cost comparison of anterior cruciate ligament reconstruction: autograft versus allograft. Arthroscopy 2005;21(7):786–90.

[46] Brown CH Jr, Carson EW. Revision anterior cruciate ligament surgery. Clin Sports Med 1999;18:109–71.

[47] Carson EW, Anisko EM, Restrepo C, et al. Revision anterior cruciate ligament reconstruction: etiology of failures and clinical results. J Knee Surg 2004;17:127–32.

[48] Ferrari JD, Bush-Joseph CA, Bach BR Jr. Arthroscopically assisted ACL reconstruction using patellar tendon substitution via endoscopic technique. In: Bach B, editor, ACL surgical techniques: techniques in orthopaedics, vol. 13. New York: Lippincott-Raven; 1998. p. 262–74.

[49] Delcogliano A, Franzese S, Branca A, et al. Light and scan electron microscopic analysis of Cyclops syndrome: etiopathogenic hypothesis and technical solutions. Knee Surg Sports Tramatol Arthrosc 1996;4:194–9.

[50] Delince P, Krallis P, Descamps PY, et al. Different aspects of the Cyclops lesion following anterior cruciate ligament reconstruction: a multifactorial etiopathogenesis. Arthroscopy 1998;14:869–76.

[51] Jackson DW, Schaefer RK. Cyclops syndrome: loss of extension following intra-articular anterior cruciate ligament reconstruction. Arthroscopy 1990;6:171–8.

[52] Marzo JM, Bowen MK, Warren RF, et al. Intraarticular fibrous nodule as a cause of loss of extension following anterior cruciate ligament reconstrucion. Arthroscopy 1992;8:10–8.
[53] Miller MD, Hinkin DT. The "N + 7 rule" for tibial tunnel placement in endoscopic anterior cruciate ligament reconstruction". Arthroscopy 1996;12:124–6.
[54] Olszewski AD, Miller MD, Ritchie JR. Ideal tibial tunnel length for endoscopic anterior cruciate ligament reconstruction. Arthroscopy 1998;14:9–14.
[55] Howell SM, Clark JA. Tibial tunnel placement in anterior cruciate ligament reconstructions and graft impingement. Clin Orthop Relat Res 1992;283:187–95.
[56] Jackson DW, Schaefer RK. Tibial tunnel placement in ACL reconstruction. Arthroscopy 1990;10:124–31.
[57] Morgan CD, Kalman VR, Grawl DM. Definitive landmarks for reproducible tibial tunnel placement in anterior cruciate ligament reconstruction. Arthroscopy 1995;11:275–88.
[58] Kurosaka M, Yoshiya S, Andrish J. A biomechanical comparison of different surgical techniques of graft fixation in anterior cruciate ligament reconstruction. Am J Sports Med 1987;15:225–9.
[59] Hackl W, Benedetto KP, Hoser C, et al. Is screw divergence in femoral bone-tendon-bone graft fixation avoidable in anterior cruciate ligament reconstruction using a single-incision technique? A radiographically controlled cadaver study. Arthroscopy 2000;16:640–7.
[60] Lemos MJ, Jackson DW, Lee TQ, et al. Assessment of initial fixation of endoscopic interference screws with divergent and parallel placement. Arthroscopy 1995;11:37–41.
[61] Pierz K, Baltz M, Fulkerson J. The effect of Kurosaka screw divergence on the holding strength of bone-tendon-bone grafts. Am J Sports Med 1995;23:332–5.
[62] Hardin GT, Bach BR Jr, Bush-Joseph CA, et al. Endoscopic single-incision anterior cruciate ligament reconstruction using patellar tendon autograft: surgical technique. J Knee Surg 2003;16(3):135–44.
[63] Rupp S, Seil R, Krauss P, et al. Cortical versus cancellous interference fixation for bone-patellar tendon-bone grafts. Arthroscopy 1998;14(5):484–8.
[64] Verma N, Noerdlinger MA, Hallab N, et al. Effects of graft rotation on initial biomechanical failure characteristics of bone-patellar tendon-bone constructs. Am J Sports Med 2003;(31):708–13.
[65] Berkson E, Lee GH, Kumar A, et al. The effect of cyclic loading on rotated bone-tendon-bone anterior cruciate ligament graft constructs. Am J Sports Med 2006;34:1442–9.
[66] Verma NN, Dennis MG, Carreira DS, et al. Preliminary clinical results of two techniques for addressing graft tunnel mismatch in endoscopic anterior cruciate ligament reconstruction. J Knee Surg 2005;18:1–9.
[67] Novak PJ, Wexler GM, Williams JS, et al. Comparison of screw post fixation and free bone block interference fixation for anterior cruciate ligament soft tissue grafts: biomechanical considerations. Arthroscopy 1996;12(4):470–3.
[68] Bach BR Jr. Revision ACL reconstruction: indications and technique. In: Miller MD, Cole BJ, editors. Textbook of arthroscopy. Philadelphia: Elsevier; 2004. p. 675–86.
[69] Charlick DA, Caborn DNM. Technical note: alternative soft-tissue graft preparation technique for cruciate ligament reconstruction. Arthroscopy 2000;16(8):20e.
[70] Brand J Jr, Weiler A, Caborn DNM, et al. Graft fixation in cruciate ligament reconstruction. Am J Sports Med 2000;28(5):761–74.
[71] West RV, Harner CD. Graft selection in anterior cruciate ligament reconstruction. J Am Acad Orthop Surg 2005;13(3):197–207.
[72] Zamorano DP, Gold SM. Reverse Achilles tendon allograft technique for anterior cruciate ligament reconstruction. Arthroscopy 2005;21(6):769e1–3.

Clin Sports Med 26 (2007) 625–637

CLINICS IN SPORTS MEDICINE

LSEVIER
AUNDERS

Freeze-Dried Allografts for Anterior Cruciate Ligament Reconstruction

Mahir Mahirogullari, MD[a,b], Cristin M. Ferguson, MD[b],
Patrick W. Whitlock, MD, PhD[b], Kathryne J. Stabile, MD, MS[b],
Gary G. Poehling, MD[b,*]

[a]Department of Orthopaedic Surgery, GATA Haydarpasa Training Hospital,
Uskudar Istanbul 34668, Turkey
[b]Department of Orthopaedic Surgery, Wake Forest University School of Medicine,
Medical Center Boulevard, 131 Miller St., Winston-Salem, NC 27157, USA

The anterior cruciate ligament (ACL) continues to be the most frequently disrupted ligament of the knee and is an injury commonly encountered by the orthopaedic surgeon [1–3]. Reconstruction of the ACL is intended to restore stability, improve function, and avoid long-term degenerative problems. Primary ACL reconstruction traditionally has been done using autogenous tissues because of the high success rate [4–7], high tissue compatibility with nonexistent immunogenicity, and the absence of the risk of disease transmission. Many surgeons continue to favor the use of bone-patellar tendon-bone (BPTB) or hamstring autograft, but several drawbacks associated with the use of autograft patellar tendon have been noted, primarily regarding donor-site morbidity with associated extensor mechanism problems. Significant quadriceps weakness was documented in 18% to 65% of patients as long as 2 years after ACL reconstruction [8,9]. Other complications associated with BPTB ACL reconstructions include joint stiffness [10], flexion contracture [9], difficulty with kneeling and knee extension [8], and patellar fracture [11]. Some studies also indicate that patellofemoral pain and concomitant crepitus to be a significant problem, occurring in as many as 80% of patients [8,9,12]. For hamstring autograft, concerns about persistent operative-side hamstring atrophy with flexion and rotational strength deficits have been raised [13–16], despite comparable patient satisfaction levels [17]. Concerns of tissue quality and availability are present in all autograft situations.

This experience has led to the use of alternative graft sources. Human allografts offer a functional substitute, with stability and clinical outcomes similar

*Corresponding author. Department of Orthopaedic Surgery, Wake Forest University School of Medicine, Medical Center Boulevard, 131 Miller St., Winston-Salem, NC 27157. E-mail address: poehling@wfubmc.edu (G.G. Poehling).

0278-5919/07/$ – see front matter
doi:10.1016/j.csm.2007.06.011

to those achieved with autografts while minimizing the problems of donor-site morbidity [3,18–22]. BPTB, Achilles tendon, tibialis tendon, fascia lata, and hamstring tendon allografts are among the main allografts used for ACL reconstruction. Allografts are useful in ACL reconstruction because of their overall availability and obvious lack of donor-site morbidity. Several studies have found allograft ACL reconstruction to be a sound alternative to autograft reconstruction [23–25], with no significant differences in symptoms, activity level, functional outcomes, or results on physical examination [18,26]. Allograft tissues have several advantages, including shorter operative and anesthetic time, better cosmesis, availability of larger grafts, lower incidence of postoperative arthrofibrosis, and, most important, no donor-site morbidity [3,27–31].

ALLOGRAFT PROCESSING

Allograft tendons are available in several forms. Fresh, fresh-frozen, cryopreserved, and freeze-dried are the most popular. Cryopreservation, a process of controlled-rate freezing with extraction of cellular water by means of dimethylsulfoxide and glycerol, is one method used for preserving menisci and ligaments at some tissue banks. In a typical cryopreservation process grafts initially are cooled to $0°C$ and are processed within 48 hours of donor death. After decontamination with antimicrobial solutions, allografts are subjected to controlled-rate freezing to $-135°C$ and are packed in a cryoprotectant solution. Cryopreserved grafts can be stored at $-196°C$ for as long as 10 years [21,22]. The increased storage costs prohibit the widespread use of cryopreserved grafts; other, less expensive techniques seem to have similar success rates [21,27]. Deep-freezing is the simplest and most common method of ligament and meniscus allograft storage. After recovery, the graft may be frozen, pending the results of donor screening and testing, after which it is thawed and processed. Freezing to $-80°C$ is typical for frozen storage. The graft then can be stored for 3 to 5 years.

Freeze-drying of human allografts for ACL surgery is less common. Although the process was described before World War II, it was not applied to human tissues until 1951 when Kreuz and colleagues [32] described the clinical transplantation of freeze-dried bone. The practice of using stored, freeze-dried tissue as a substitute for injured tissue has been developed over many years [33–38]. The freeze-drying procedures are more complicated and lengthier than those for deep-freezing. The graft is procured under sterile conditions and then is frozen. Once the tissue has passed the initial tests, physical débridement occurs, which includes ethanol treatment, antibiotic soaks, and blood/lipid removal. The tissue finally is preserved through freeze-drying, in which the tissue is refrozen and lyophilized to a residual moisture of less than 5%. Once cultures obtained during débridement are cleared, and serologic assays are negative, the allograft is released for use [22,28]. The graft then can be packaged and stored at room temperature for 3 to 5 years. Rehydration of freeze-dried ligament grafts requires a minimum of 30 minutes before transplantation.

All allografts should come with the highest possible assurance that they are free of pathogens. Aseptic processing is the most common method of allograft preparation in the United States today [22]. Aseptic processing refers to methods used by a manufacturer to avoid adding contamination to a product. The most common method of minimizing allograft contamination is to adhere to sterile techniques during harvest, transport, and processing [21]. The tissues are soaked in antibiotic solution at 4°C for at least 1 hour, and multiple cultures are obtained during processing. Low-dose gamma radiation (< 2.0 mrad) may be used as an adjunct to help with sterilization while maintaining the mechanical properties of the graft, but radiation at this level does not eliminate HIV and hepatitis viruses [39,40]. Haut and Powlison [41] have examined the possible interaction of multiple sterilization treatments. They evaluated the effect of a sequence of irradiating and freeze-drying on the biomechanical properties of human BPTB preparations. They found significant decreases in the modulus and strength if the specimens were lyophilized before irradiation. No significant effect was noted for specimens lyophilized after irradiation. Rihn and colleagues [42] compared the clinical outcome of ACL reconstruction with irradiated allograft versus autograft. They found that the patients undergoing ACL reconstruction with irradiated allograft BPTB had clinical outcomes similar to those reconstructed with autograft BPTB. They suggested that irradiation could be used to help sterilize BPTB allograft without adversely affecting clinical outcome. The authors' preferred allograft is freeze-dried Achilles tendon that is not irradiated or exposed to low levels of irradiation (< 1.8 mrad) before the lyophilization process.

FREEZE-DRIED ALLOGRAFTS: MECHANICAL PROPERTIES

Because irradiation processing of allografts affects the mechanical properties of tissue, the process of lyophilization also has potential to impact the mechanical properties of allografts before implantation. For soft tissue allografts, Thomas and Gresham [43] found that freeze-dried fascia lata grafts are initially equal in strength to fresh allograft tissue. Comparison of implanted freeze-dried flexor tendon allografts with autografts in a dog flexor tendon repair model showed that the allograft and autograft tissue had similar mechanical properties at 3 and 6 months after implantation. Both were approximately one third the strength of normal tendon. Similar histology of autograft and allograft tendons was observed [38]. Direct studies of the preimplantation of bone containing freeze-dried ACL allografts have not been performed. Lyophilization has been shown to reduce the ultimate strength and stiffness of cancellous bone after rehydration by 18.9% and 20%, respectively [44]. This finding suggests that the mechanical properties of lyophilized allograft BPTB at the bone–tunnel interface may be inferior to those of fresh-frozen allograft. Further studies are warranted to test this hypothesis as well as the mechanical properties of the bone–tendon interface after lyophilization of BPTB allograft.

FREEZE-DRIED ALLOGRAFTS: BIOLOGIC INCORPORATION, IMMUNOGENICITY, AND DISEASE TRANSMISSION

Different studies have shown that both autograft and fresh-frozen allografts undergo a process of peripheral synovialization, central ischemic necrosis, revascularization, cellular proliferation and graft repopulation, and eventual ligament engraftment [45–50]. Some studies have shown that the biologic incorporation and remodeling processes are slower in allografts than in autogenous grafts [21,51–54]. Both autografts and allografts are weaker during the incorporation phase with lower maximum load-to-failure when compared with normal tissue, but the effect is more pronounced in allografts [47,55]. Even with observations of remodeling processes extending past 6-, 12-, and even 18-months, however, there are no published reports of studies indicating an increased risk of failure of allograft constructs.

Few studies specifically have examined the biologic incorporation of freeze-dried allografts. Biopsy samples were obtained arthroscopically from the midportion of the ACL grafts of 21 patients who had undergone freeze-dried nonirradiated fascia lata allograft and studied at time points ranging from 3 to 20 months postoperatively. Arthroscopically, all grafts appeared fully synovialized. Subjectively, the grafts followed a progression of early peripheral synovialization and active fibroplasia (cellular proliferation) toward the central areas of the graft, followed by intermediate fibroplasia with increased collagen fiber deposition. After 6 months, there was progressive maturation of the connective tissue toward normal ACL with decreased cellularity, vascularity, and fibroplasia. Progression of histologic maturity as gauged by polarization of collagen fibers continued through 20 months, suggesting continued progression of maturation and remodeling of the collagen fibers. Close examination of the numeric data suggests that the polarization changes plateau between 9 and 13 months, indicating the nearly final maturation stage [56]. A report of a case 2.5 years after freeze-dried Achilles tendon allograft ACL reconstruction showed histologic attachment of the allograft ligament to bone through Sharpey's fiber attachments, full graft maturation with normal cellularity, and crimp pattern [28]. This report suggests that aseptically processed freeze-dried allograft follows a progression of biologic incorporation and remodeling similar to that of fresh-frozen allograft constructs, but further study is needed to understand better the differences in the biologic and temporal progression and strength properties of autograft and allograft (freeze-dried versus fresh-frozen) constructs.

Immunogenicity properties of transplanted allografts are postulated to affect host inflammatory response and allograft incorporation. Fresh bone allografts have been reported to be the most immunogenic, frozen grafts to be less immunogenic, and freeze-dried allografts to be the least immunogenic [57,58]. The changes in the properties and makeup of freeze-dried biologic material have been attributed to the alterations in protein configurations or the blocking of hydrophilic sites of proteins by oxidation associated with drying. The alterations caused by freeze-drying probably are responsible for the reduction in the antigenicity [59]. The immunogenicity of skeletal tissues is diminished if the grafts are frozen before transplantation. The immunogenicity resulting from histocompatibility antigens are reduced further if the allografts are freeze-dried [57,59], indicating that freeze-dried constructs might be an attractive source of ACL allografts. Future studies are indicated to examine more closely the impact and mechanism of immunogenicity reactions on the progression and success of biologic incorporation.

The issue of disease transmission with transfusions and implanted allograft tissue has come to the forefront over the last 20 years, with concerns primarily regarding the transmission of hepatitis and HIV. HIV and hepatitis C transmission has occurred through the transplantation of allograft bone and tendon. As of 1995, there were two documented cases of HIV-infected tissue, one case of hepatitis B–infected tissue, and three cases of hepatitis C–infected donor tissue used for transplantation of musculoskeletal allografts, resulting in several cases of disease transmission [60]. In 1985 [61], 58 bone and soft tissue allografts and organs were obtained from a single infected donor and a single tissue bank. A number of recipients became HIV positive 5 years later, and retrospective polymerase chain-reaction testing on archived tissue identified the donor as HIV positive. Four patients received fresh-frozen allografts, and three of these patients tested positive for HIV. None of the 42 recipients of freeze-dried grafts obtained from this donor became infected with HIV [61]. After a controlled laboratory study, however, Crawford and colleagues [40] reported that freeze-drying should not be relied on to inactivate infectious retrovirus in systemically infected musculoskeletal allografts. According to the last published statistics of the American Association of Tissue Banks, more than 2 million musculoskeletal allografts have been distributed to surgeons for transplantation into patients during the past 5 years, with no documented incident of a viral infectious disease transmission caused by an allograft.

BASIC SCIENCE OUTCOMES: FREEZE-DRIED BONE-PATELLAR TENDON-BONE AND SOFT TISSUE TENDON

In 1983, Webster and Werner [37,38] used freeze-dried flexor tendons in ACL reconstruction in dogs. Examination after 8 months showed that the allografts were repopulated by host cells. They reported that the mechanical properties of allograft were similar to those of autograft constructs but were inferior to native ACL. Curtis and colleagues [62] reconstructed the ACL with freeze-dried fascia lata allografts in dogs. They found no biologic incompatibility or immune response. The failure strength of the allograft side was 67% of the contralateral side at the 6-month evaluation. This finding can be compared with fresh-frozen patellar tendon allografts, which reached 35% of the strength of the normal ACL in another dog study [50]. In 1987, Jackson and colleagues [47,63,64] studied 11 freeze-dried ethylene oxide (EO)–sterilized ACL BPTB allografts in a goat model. At 12 months, they found significantly greater anteroposterior laxity and less stiffness and strength than in controls and normal histology of healing, with absence of immune reaction and normal-appearing vascularity.

Further studies of EO-sterilized freeze-dried allografts have raised concerns about safety and function. The clinical study by Jackson and colleagues [65] raises the question of whether EO causes intra-articular synovial and immune reactions. Of 109 patients who underwent ACL reconstruction with a freeze-dried, EO-sterilized, BPTB allograft, 7 patients (6.4%) developed a persistent intra-articular reaction. The reaction was characterized by persistent synovial effusion with collagenous particulates and cellular inflammatory response. There was no direct evidence of toxicity with EO or its by-products, but the reactions resolved with removal of the EO-sterilized soft tissue grafts. Using gas chromatography, the investigators examined one of the seven grafts that was removed and measured high levels of ethylene chlorohydrin. It was unclear whether the EO-sterilized grafts caused the synovitis reaction. Human leukocyte antigen conversion was noted in three of the seven allografts recipients. A study by Roberts and colleagues [66] found complete dissolution of the graft on repeat surgery in 8 of 36 patients (22%) who received freeze-dried EO-sterilized BPTB allografts. The exact cause of graft dissolution was unclear, but the authors agreed with Jackson and colleagues that the most probable cause of graft failure was EO and its byproducts. Butler and colleagues [67], Gibbons and colleagues [68], and Paulos and colleagues [69] evaluated the mechanical properties of allografts before and after sterilization and preservation and also concluded that EO gas sterilization is not an acceptable procedure.

In summary, basic science and animal studies suggest that, in the absence of EO sterilization, freeze-dried allografts are an allograft tissue source at least equivalent to fresh-frozen allograft constructs. Further animal studies comparing functional, mechanical, and biologic incorporation results among equivalent freeze-dried and fresh-frozen allograft and autograft constructs are warranted to improve the understanding of ACL reconstruction techniques.

CLINICAL OUTCOMES: FREEZE-DRIED ALLOGRAFT CONSTRUCTS

The first large clinical study of freeze-dried allograft for ACL reconstruction reviewed the outcome of 23 cases of arthroscopic ACL reconstruction using freeze-dried Achilles allograft tendons in a prospective study [70]. They reported that all patients with at least 20 months follow-up resumed their preinjury activity levels. Only one patient experienced worsening of KT-1000 (MEDmetric Corporation, San Diego, California) arthrometer readings and had a positive pivot-shift test result. No adverse outcomes were observed. Noyes and colleagues [24] performed ACL reconstruction with fresh-frozen BPTB and freeze-dried fascia lata allograft. They found no significant differences between patients who had the two different grafts. One failure was a fascia lata graft. Eighteen of the 22 freeze-dried fascia lata grafts had been sterilized with EO. Indelicato and colleagues [71] compared clinical outcomes of freeze-dried and fresh-frozen allograft tissue used as a substitute for a ruptured ACL. They used 21 parameters in their comparison of fresh-frozen and freeze-dried

BPTB and found a significant difference in only 3 of the 21 parameters evaluated. They concluded that there was no clinical evidence of rejection phenomena in either group. Meyers and colleagues [72] used freeze-dried allografts for arthroscopic intra-articular ACL reconstructions. They stated that they were encouraged by the clinical and arthroscopic findings using this technique. Levitt and colleagues [23] treated ACL-deficient knees with freeze-dried or fresh-frozen BPTB and Achilles allograft (with attached bone plug). They found that 80% of all patients were satisfied. No significant difference was noted between Achilles and patellar tendon allografts and between fresh-frozen and freeze-dried grafts. They concluded that allograft reconstruction of a deficient ACL could be performed successfully.

At the Department of Orthopaedic Surgery at Wake Forest University School of Medicine, 1270 ACL-deficient knees were operated on using Achilles freeze-dried allograft by the same senior surgeon (GGP) between 1985 and 2005. The authors know of no cases of disease transmission or any allograft rejection reactions. They performed a prospective study to compare outcomes of primary ACL reconstruction with either freeze-dried Achilles tendon allograft with soft-tissue fixation or standard BPTB autograft with interference screw fixation [3]. The results included 41 patients who underwent soft tissue allograft reconstruction and 118 patients who underwent autograft BPTB reconstruction. Patients were evaluated preoperatively and postoperatively at 1 to 2 weeks, 6 weeks, 3 months, 6 months, and then annually for 5 years. Objective measures of outcome included KT-1000 measurements, range of motion, ligamentous integrity, thigh atrophy, and International Knee Documentation Committee score. Subjective evaluations included patient completion of five questionnaires documenting functional status, pain, and health-related quality of life. Patient assessment of function and symptoms showed that a higher proportion of patients reported normal or nearly normal knee function in the allograft group than in the autograft group at 3 months. Fewer activity limitations at 6 weeks, 3 months, and 6 months were reported by patients receiving freeze-dried allograft than by those receiving BPTB autograft. After reconstruction, the allograft group displayed a trend toward more laxity in KT-1000 measurements at all time points than did the autograft group (mean, 3.0 mm versus 2.8 mm; $P = .0520$). These measurements decreased over time for both groups. Both groups of patients achieved similar long-term clinical outcomes. Overall, the allograft patients reported better function at 1 week, 3 months, and 1 year and fewer activity limitations throughout the follow-up period. Previous studies have failed to include data on pain from the short-term postoperative period. Analysis of the study data showed that allograft patients reported significantly less pain than autograft patients within the first 3 months after surgery. Patients who had allografts also reported less frequent pain during ambulation as assessed by the Knee Pain Questionnaire at 6 months and less severe pain on ambulation at 6 months and 1 year than patients who had autografts [3]. An expected reduction in postoperative pain associated with the allograft reconstruction procedure may be a significant factor for patients who desire a less painful recovery and a quicker return to work [3].

The authors also compared the economic costs associated with ACL reconstruction using either BPTB autograft or freeze-dried Achilles allograft [73]. A total of 122 patients who had ACL-deficient knees undergoing surgical reconstruction using either BPTB autograft (n = 86) or freeze-dried Achilles tendon allograft (n = 37) were analyzed. Groups were compared with respect to hospital charge data obtained from the billing department. The mean hospital charge for ACL reconstruction was $4622 for freeze-dried allograft and $5694 for autograft ($P < .0001$). Differences included increased operating room time and a greater likelihood of overnight hospitalization for autograft procedures. The authors found that freeze-dried allograft reconstruction of the ACL was significantly less costly than autograft BPTB reconstruction [73].

Many of the original studies of freeze-dried allograft using soft tissue grafts were performed before current advanced arthroscopy techniques and advanced soft tissue fixation devices. The senior author has employed less commonly used devices for femoral and tibial soft tissue graft fixation than the majority in the field, and the emphasis on the importance of anatomic graft placement has been maintained over the years. Even with less rigid fixation devices and absence of aperture fixation (which may not be essential for clinical success) [74], the use of aseptically processed freeze-dried soft tissue allograft has produced consistently positive clinical functional outcomes without problematic adverse reactions or outcomes.

FREEZE-DRIED ALLOGRAFT: SUMMARY OF ADVANTAGES AND DISADVANTAGES

Although less commonly reported, freeze-dried allografts represent a viable and functional alternative to fresh-frozen allograft and autograft constructs. Freeze-dried soft tissue allograft constructs have many advantages. Initial mechanical properties of freeze-dried soft tissue allografts are maintained after lyophilization processing. Freeze-dried constructs that include bone may be less ideal because the structural properties of bone decline during lyophilization. Biologically, freeze-dried allografts offer the potential for lower immunogenicity reactions than encountered with fresh-frozen constructs and approach the limited immune response of autograft constructs. Further basic science studies are necessary to understand the immunologic aspects of the biologic process of graft incorporation. Although freeze-drying has not been shown to eliminate the transmission of viral diseases in basic science studies, there have been no clinical reports of the transmission of viral disease through freeze-dried allograft tissues obtained from known individuals to be infected. Freeze-drying allows storage at room temperatures for 3 to 5 years. Clinical studies of freeze-dried allograft constructs without EO sterilization have shown results equivalent to those with fresh-frozen allograft constructs [3]. Further basic science and clinical studies are indicated to compare directly the results of freeze-dried allograft soft tissue constructs with fresh-frozen allograft and autograft soft tissue constructs, maintaining constant operative technique parameters.

FUTURE DIRECTIONS: ANTERIOR CRUCIATE LIGAMENT ALLOGRAFT

Although there is sufficient evidence to support their use, freeze-dried allografts have not been widely used in the United States. This lack of use does not correlate with the published scientific literature supporting the excellent functional outcomes achieved with freeze-dried allografts. Compared with fresh-frozen allografts, freeze-dried allografts are easy to use, readily available, and cost effective. Based on the Department of Orthopaedic Surgery at Wake Forest University School of Medicine's extensive experience with freeze-dried allografts, the authors expect that these grafts will be used with increasing frequency in the future, especially when combined with current and future tissue-engineering technologies.

An ideal graft is one that has very little donor-site morbidity, no inflammatory potential or host immune response, is biocompatible in vitro and in vivo, has no disease transmission, and has optimal biologic incorporation with biomechanics equivalent to the intact ACL. At present, this graft does not exist; it is hoped that tissue engineering and future technologies will realize this ideal graft more closely than do the current standard autograft and allograft options.

Freeze-dried allografts are considered acellular and therefore devoid of living or intact antigen-presenting cells. Several authors even have concluded that

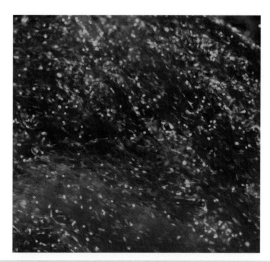

Fig. 1. Fluorescent picture showing surface image of an ACL scaffold derived from human Achilles tendon allograft 48 hours after seeding with murine fibroblasts (original magnification × 4). Fibroblasts are expressing green fluorescent protein. Homogenous cell density and penetration are clearly evident in this image. (*Courtesy of* P.W. Whitlock, MD, PhD, Winston-Salem, NC.)

they are incapable of eliciting a detectable immune response [75]. This conclusion is supported further by a lack of histologic evidence of immunologic rejection in allografts retrieved from patients 20 days to 10 years after transplantation [76]. Because of their minimal inflammatory potential, freeze-dried allografts are more likely to be a better starting material than fresh-frozen tissue for use in tissue-engineering scaffold development. Although the lyophilization process can be considered an improved method for allograft processing, this technique is far from optimal. The authors' initial research investigations indicate that the microarchitecture of freeze-dried allografts can be modified structurally through tissue-engineering techniques to improve further host cell infiltration, attachment, and growth (**Fig. 1**). Such improvements can lead to more rapid engraftment and incorporation, increased functional regeneration with strength characteristics closer to intact ACL, and therefore even more favorable clinical outcomes than currently achieved. With more rapid and complete biologic incorporation using engineered allograft tissues, we may someday provide patients with a stronger reconstruction and a more rapid return to function and sport than observed with current autograft and allograft constructs.

References

[1] Eriksson E. Reconstruction of the anterior cruciate ligament. Orthop Clin North Am 1976;7(1):167–79.
[2] Johnson RJ, Beynnon BD, Nichols CE, et al. The treatment of injuries of the anterior cruciate ligament. J Bone Joint Surg Am 1992;74(1):140–51.
[3] Poehling GG, Curl WW, Lee CA, et al. Analysis of outcomes of anterior cruciate ligament repair with 5-year follow-up: allograft versus autograft. Arthroscopy 2005;21(7):774–85.
[4] Aglietti P, Buzzi R, Zaccherotti G, et al. Patellar tendon versus doubled semitendinosus and gracilis tendons for anterior cruciate ligament reconstruction. Am J Sports Med 1994;22(2): 211–7 [discussion: 217–8].
[5] Goradia VK, Grana WA. A comparison of outcomes at 2 to 6 years after acute and chronic anterior cruciate ligament reconstructions using hamstring tendon grafts. Arthroscopy 2001;17(4):383–92.
[6] Jomha NM, Pinczewski LA, Clingeleffer A, et al. Arthroscopic reconstruction of the anterior cruciate ligament with patellar-tendon autograft and interference screw fixation. The results at seven years. J Bone Joint Surg Br 1999;81(5):775–9.
[7] Shelbourne KD, Urch SE. Primary anterior cruciate ligament reconstruction using the contralateral autogenous patellar tendon. Am J Sports Med 2000;28(5):651–8.
[8] Rosenberg TD, Franklin JL, Baldwin GN, et al. Extensor mechanism function after patellar tendon graft harvest for anterior cruciate ligament reconstruction. Am J Sports Med 1992;20(5):519–25, [discussion: 525–6].
[9] Sachs RA, Daniel DM, Stone ML, et al. Patellofemoral problems after anterior cruciate ligament reconstruction. Am J Sports Med 1989;17(6):760–5.
[10] Miller MD, Harner CD. The use of allograft. Techniques and results. Clin Sports Med 1993;12(4):757–70.
[11] Simonian PT, Mann FA, Mandt PR. Indirect forces and patella fracture after anterior cruciate ligament reconstruction with the patellar ligament. Case report. Am J Knee Surg 1995;8(2): 60–4 [discussion: 64–5].
[12] Svensson M, Kartus J, Ejerhed L, et al. Does the patellar tendon normalize after harvesting its central third?: a prospective long-term MRI study. Am J Sports Med 2004;32(1):34–8.

[13] Burks RT, Crim J, Fink BP, et al. The effects of semitendinosus and gracilis harvest in anterior cruciate ligament reconstruction. Arthroscopy 2005;21(10):1177–85.

[14] Adachi N, Ochi M, Uchio Y, et al. Harvesting hamstring tendons for ACL reconstruction influences postoperative hamstring muscle performance. Arch Orthop Trauma Surg 2003;123(9):460–5.

[15] Nakamura N, Horibe S, Sasaki S, et al. Evaluation of active knee flexion and hamstring strength after anterior cruciate ligament reconstruction using hamstring tendons. Arthroscopy 2002;18(6):598–602.

[16] Armour T, Forwell L, Litchfield R, et al. Isokinetic evaluation of internal/external tibial rotation strength after the use of hamstring tendons for anterior cruciate ligament reconstruction. Am J Sports Med 2004;32(7):1639–43.

[17] Beynnon BD, Johnson RJ, Fleming BC, et al. Anterior cruciate ligament replacement: comparison of bone-patellar tendon-bone grafts with two-strand hamstring grafts. A prospective, randomized study. J Bone Joint Surg Am 2002;84-A(9):1503–13.

[18] Harner CD, Olson E, Irrgang JJ, et al. Allograft versus autograft anterior cruciate ligament reconstruction: 3- to 5-year outcome. Clin Orthop Relat Res 1996;(324):134–44.

[19] Lephart SM, Kocher MS, Harner CD, et al. Quadriceps strength and functional capacity after anterior cruciate ligament reconstruction. Patellar tendon autograft versus allograft. Am J Sports Med 1993;21(5):738–43.

[20] Saddemi SR, Frogameni AD, Fenton PJ, et al. Comparison of perioperative morbidity of anterior cruciate ligament autografts versus allografts. Arthroscopy 1993;9(5):519–24.

[21] Shelton WR, Treacy SH, Dukes AD, et al. Use of allografts in knee reconstruction: II. Surgical considerations. J Am Acad Orthop Surg 1998;6(3):169–75.

[22] Vangsness CT Jr, Garcia IA, Mills CR, et al. Allograft transplantation in the knee: tissue regulation, procurement, processing, and sterilization. Am J Sports Med 2003;31(3):474–81.

[23] Levitt RL, Malinin T, Posada A, et al. Reconstruction of anterior cruciate ligaments with bone-patellar tendon-bone and Achilles tendon allografts. Clin Orthop Relat Res 1994;(303): 67–78.

[24] Noyes FR, Barber SD, Mangine RE. Bone-patellar ligament-bone and fascia lata allografts for reconstruction of the anterior cruciate ligament. J Bone Joint Surg Am 1990;72(8): 1125–36.

[25] Noyes FR, Barber-Westin SD. Reconstruction of the anterior cruciate ligament with human allograft. Comparison of early and later results. J Bone Joint Surg Am 1996;78(4): 524–37.

[26] Shelton WR, Papendick L, Dukes AD. Autograft versus allograft anterior cruciate ligament reconstruction. Arthroscopy 1997;13(4):446–9.

[27] Barbour SA, King W. The safe and effective use of allograft tissue—an update. Am J Sports Med 2003;31(5):791–7.

[28] Lee CA, Meyer JV, Shilt JS, et al. Allograft maturation in anterior cruciate ligament reconstruction. Arthroscopy 2004;20(Suppl 2):46–9.

[29] McGuire DA. Should allografts be used for routine anterior cruciate ligament reconstructions? Yes, allografts should be used in routine ACL reconstruction. Arthroscopy 2003;19(4): 421–4.

[30] Shino K, Inoue M, Horibe S, et al. Maturation of allograft tendons transplanted into the knee. An arthroscopic and histological study. J Bone Joint Surg Br 1988;70(4):556–60.

[31] Shino K, Nakagawa S, Inoue M, et al. Deterioration of patellofemoral articular surfaces after anterior cruciate ligament reconstruction. Am J Sports Med 1993;21(2):206–11.

[32] Kreuz FP, Hyatt GW, Turner TC, et al. The preservation and clinical use of freeze-dried bone. J Bone Joint Surg Am 1951;33-A(4):863–72, [passim].

[33] Andreeff I, Dimoff G, Metschkarski S. A comparative experimental study on transplantation of autogenous and homogenous tendon tissue. Acta Orthop Scand 1967;38(1):35–44.

[34] Gresham RB. Freeze-drying of human tissue for clinical use. Cryobiology 1964;1(2): 150–6.

[35] Gresham RB. The freeze-dried cortical bone homograft: a roentgenographic and histologic evaluation. Clin Orthop Relat Res 1964;37:194–201.

[36] Hyatt GW, Wilber MC. The storage of human tissues for surgical use. Postgrad Med J 1959;35(404):338–43.

[37] Webster DA, Werner FW. Freeze-dried flexor tendons in anterior cruciate ligament reconstruction. Clin Orthop Relat Res 1983;(181):238–43.

[38] Webster DA, Werner FW. Mechanical and functional properties of implanted freeze-dried flexor tendons. Clin Orthop Relat Res 1983;(180):301–9.

[39] Fideler BM, Vangsness CT Jr, Lu B, et al. Gamma irradiation: effects on biomechanical properties of human bone-patellar tendon-bone allografts. Am J Sports Med 1995;23(5):643–6.

[40] Crawford C, Kainer M, Jernigan D, et al. Investigation of postoperative allograft-associated infections in patients who underwent musculoskeletal allograft implantation. Clin Infect Dis 2005;41(2):195–200.

[41] Haut RC, Powlison AC. The effects of test environment and cyclic stretching on the failure properties of human patellar tendons. J Orthop Res 1990;8(4):532–40.

[42] Rihn JA, Irrgang JJ, Chhabra A, et al. Does irradiation affect the clinical outcome of patellar tendon allograft ACL reconstruction? Knee Surg Sports Traumatol Arthrosc 2006;14(9): 885–96.

[43] Thomas ED, Gresham RB. Comparative tensile strength study of fresh, frozen, and freeze-dried human fascia lata. Surg Forum 1963;14:442–3.

[44] Cornu O, Banse X, Docquier PL, et al. Effect of freeze-drying and gamma irradiation on the mechanical properties of human cancellous bone. J Orthop Res 2000;18(3):426–31.

[45] Arnoczky SP, Warren RF, Ashlock MA. Replacement of the anterior cruciate ligament using a patellar tendon allograft. An experimental study. J Bone Joint Surg Am 1986;68(3): 376–85.

[46] Goertzen M, Dellmann A, Gruber J, et al. Anterior cruciate ligament allograft transplantation for intraarticular ligamentous reconstruction. Arch Orthop Trauma Surg 1992;111(5): 273–9.

[47] Jackson DW, Grood ES, Arnoczky SP, et al. Preliminary studies in a goat model. Am J Sports Med 1987;15(4):295–303.

[48] Mologne TS, Friedman MJ. Graft options for ACL reconstruction. Am J Orthop 2000;29(11):845–53.

[49] Nikolaou PK, Seaber AV, Glisson RR, et al. Anterior cruciate ligament allograft transplantation. Long-term function, histology, revascularization, and operative technique. Am J Sports Med 1986;14(5):348–60.

[50] Shino K, Kawasaki T, Hirose H, et al. Replacement of the anterior cruciate ligament by an allogeneic tendon graft. An experimental study in the dog. J Bone Joint Surg Br 1984;66(5):672–81.

[51] Cordrey LJ. A comparative study of fresh autogenous and preserved homogenous tendon grafts in rabbits. J Bone Joint Surg Br 1963;45-B:182–95.

[52] Gazdag AR, Lane JM, Glaser D, et al. Alternatives to autogenous bone graft: efficacy and indications. J Am Acad Orthop Surg 1995;3(1):1–8.

[53] Jackson DW, Corsetti J, Simon TM. Biologic incorporation of allograft anterior cruciate ligament replacements. Clin Orthop Relat Res 1996;(324):126–33.

[54] Jackson DW, Kenna R, Simon TM, et al. Endoscopic ACL reconstruction. Orthopedics 1993;16(9):951–8.

[55] Drez DJ Jr, DeLee J, Holden JP, et al. A biological and biomechanical evaluation in goats. Am J Sports Med 1991;19(3):256–63.

[56] Horstman JK, Ahmadu-Suka F, Norrdin RW. Anterior cruciate ligament fascia lata allograft reconstruction: progressive histologic changes toward maturity. Arthroscopy 1993;9(5): 509–18.

[57] Friedlaender GE. Immune responses to osteochondral allografts. Current knowledge and future directions. Clin Orthop Relat Res 1983;(174):58–68.

[58] Czitrom AA, Langer F, McKee N, et al. Bone and cartilage allotransplantation. A review of 14 years of research and clinical studies. Clin Orthop Relat Res 1986;(208):141–5.

[59] Malinin T. Preparation and banking of bone and tendon allografts. In: Sherman OH, Minkoff J, editors. Arthroscopy surgery. 1st edition. Baltimore (MD): Williams&Wilkins; 1990. p. 65–85.

[60] Tomford WW. Transmission of disease through transplantation of musculoskeletal allografts. J Bone Joint Surg Am 1995;77(11):1742–54.

[61] Asselmeier MA, Caspari RB, Bottenfield S. A review of allograft processing and sterilization techniques and their role in transmission of the human immunodeficiency virus. Am J Sports Med 1993;21(2):170–5.

[62] Curtis RJ, Delee JC, Drez DJ Jr. Reconstruction of the anterior cruciate ligament with freeze dried fascia lata allografts in dogs. A preliminary report. Am J Sports Med 1985;13(6): 408–14.

[63] Jackson DW, Grood ES, Arnoczky SP, et al. Cruciate reconstruction using freeze dried anterior cruciate ligament allograft and a ligament augmentation device (LAD). An experimental study in a goat model. Am J Sports Med 1987;15(6):528–38.

[64] Jackson DW, Grood ES, Cohn BT, et al. The effects of in situ freezing on the anterior cruciate ligament. An experimental study in goats. J Bone Joint Surg Am 1991;73(2):201–13.

[65] Jackson DW, Windler GE, Simon TM. Intraarticular reaction associated with the use of freeze-dried, ethylene oxide-sterilized bone-patella tendon-bone allografts in the reconstruction of the anterior cruciate ligament. Am J Sports Med 1990;18(1):1–10 [discussion 10–1].

[66] Roberts TS, Drez D Jr, McCarthy W, et al. Two year results in thirty-six patients. Am J Sports Med 1991;19(1):35–41.

[67] Butler DL, Noyes FR, Walz KA. Biomechanics of human knee ligament allograft treatment. Transactions of Orthopaedic Research Society 1987;12:128.

[68] Gibbons MJ, Butler DL, Grood ES. Dose dependent effects of gamma irradiation on the material properties of frozen bone-patellar tendon-bone allografts. Transactions of the Orthopaedic Research Society 1989;14:513.

[69] Paulos LE, France EP, Rosenberg TD. Comparative material properties of allograft tissues for ligament replacement: effect of type, age, sterilization and preservation. Transactions of the Orthopaedic Research Society 1987;12:129.

[70] Wainer RA, Clarke TJ, Poehling GG. Arthroscopic reconstruction of the anterior cruciate ligament using allograft tendon. Arthroscopy 1988;4(3):199–205.

[71] Indelicato PA, Bittar ES, Prevot TJ, et al. Clinical comparison of freeze-dried and fresh frozen patellar tendon allografts for anterior cruciate ligament reconstruction of the knee. Am J Sports Med 1990;18(4):335–42.

[72] Meyers JF, Caspari RB, Cash JD, et al. Arthroscopic evaluation of allograft anterior cruciate ligament reconstruction. Arthroscopy 1992;8(2):157–61.

[73] Cole DW, Ginn TA, Chen GJ, et al. Cost comparison of anterior cruciate ligament reconstruction: autograft versus allograft. Arthroscopy 2005;21(7):786–90.

[74] Farmer JM, Lee CA, Curl WW, et al. Initial biomechanical properties of staple-anchor Achilles tendon allograft and interference screw bone-patellar tendon-bone autograft fixation for anterior cruciate ligament reconstruction in a cadaveric model. Arthroscopy 2006;22(10): 1040–5.

[75] Horowitz MC, Friedlaender GE. Immunologic aspects of bone transplantation. A rationale for future studies. Orthop Clin North Am 1987;18(2):227–33.

[76] Malinin TI, Levitt RL, Bashore C, et al. A study of retrieved allografts used to replace anterior cruciate ligaments. Arthroscopy 2002;18(2):163–70.

Soft Tissue Allograft and Double-Bundle Reconstruction

Samir G. Tejwani, MD[a], Wei Shen, MD, PhD[b],
Freddie H. Fu, MD, DSc(Hon), DPs(Hon)[b,*]

[a]Kaiser Permanente, Department of Orthopaedic Surgery, 9985 Sierra Avenue, Fontana, CA 92335, USA
[b]Department of Orthopaedic Surgery, University of Pittsburgh, 3471 5th Avenue, Suite 1011, Pittsburgh, PA 15213, USA

An estimated 80,000 anterior cruciate ligament (ACL) tears occur annually in the United States, with the highest incidence in individuals 15 to 25 years old who participate in pivoting sports [1]. These injuries occur by multiple mechanisms, resulting in variable patterns of rupture. The ACL is composed of two distinct functional bundles of fibers, the anteromedial (AM) and posterolateral (PL), which have been observed in fetal development as early as 16 weeks' gestation [2–6]. A thorough knowledge of ACL anatomy is critical for correct tunnel placement and successful surgical reconstruction (Figs. 1–3).

The AM and PL bundles originate from the medial aspect of the lateral femoral condyle and insert between the tibial spines. The AM bundle has an approximate length of 34 mm, originates from the anterior and proximal aspect of the femoral attachment (67 mm^2), and inserts into the AM aspect of the tibial attachment (67 mm^2). The PL bundle originates more distally on the femoral attachment (66 mm^2), inserts on the PL attachment off the tibial insertion (52 mm^2), and has an approximate length of 23 mm. Functionally, their roles are complementary, with the AM bundle tight in flexion and the PL bundle tight in extension [5,7–10]. In full knee extension the two bundles are parallel in orientation. As the knee flexes to 90°, which is the most typical position during surgery for ACL reconstruction, the origins of the two bundles on the femur change from a vertical to horizontal alignment, and the PL bundle crosses the AM bundle [4,11].

RATIONALE FOR DOUBLE-BUNDLE RECONSTRUCTION

Traditional single-bundle (SB) ACL surgical techniques have focused on reconstruction of only the AM bundle, with generally good results. A critical review

*Corresponding author. Department of Orthopaedic Surgery, University of Pittsburgh, 3471 5th Avenue, Suite 1011, Pittsburgh, PA 15213, USA. *E-mail address*: ffu@upmc.edu (F.H. Fu).

0278-5919/07/$ – see front matter
doi:10.1016/j.csm.2007.06.004

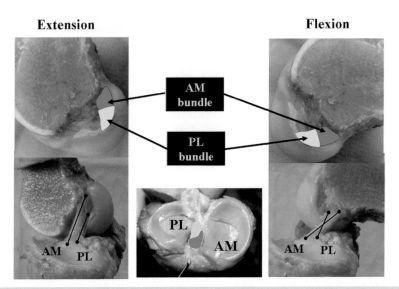

Fig. 1. Right knee: in full extension (*left panels*) the femoral insertion sites of the anteromedial (AM, *red*) and posterolateral (PL, *yellow*) bundles of the ACL are vertical. In 90° of knee flexion (*right panels*) the insertion sites are horizontal. The fibers of the two bundles are parallel in extension and cross each other as the knee is flexed. Tibial insertion sites are indicated in the region of the tibial spines (*center panel*).

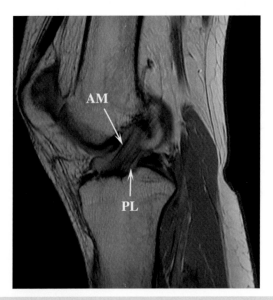

Fig. 2. Left knee: standard sagittal image demonstrating the anteromedial (AM) and posterolateral (PL) bundles of the ACL.

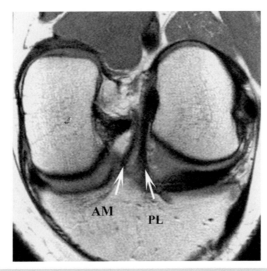

Fig. 3. Left knee: oblique coronal MRI in the plane of the ACL demonstrating the anteromedial (AM) and posterolateral (PL) bundles.

of the literature, however, shows that some patients have residual instability and pain following SB reconstruction [12–15]. In a prospective study, Fithian and colleagues [16] found radiographic evidence of degenerative changes in 90% of patients at 7 years after SB reconstruction; only 47% were able to return to their previous activity level. Kocher and colleagues [17] found a significant association between the pivot-shift test and functional outcome after SB ACL reconstruction and no correlation between the KT-1000 and Lachman tests and functional outcome, emphasizing the importance of restoring rotational stability in the knee.

Numerous biomechanical studies have been devoted to elucidating the role of the PL bundle of the ACL. The AM bundle limits anterior tibial translation through the full range of knee motion, whereas the PL bundle does so in the final 45° of extension [18]. In addition, the PL bundle tightens during internal and external rotation when the knee is near full extension and thus plays a critical role in the rotational stability of the knee [19]. In a laboratory study, Zantop and colleagues [20] found that isolated transection of the PL bundle increased anterior tibial translation at 30° of knee flexion and resulted in increased combined rotation at 0° and 30°, with or without section of the AM bundle. Woo and colleagues [21] and Yagi and colleagues [22] have demonstrated that SB ACL reconstruction of the AM bundle is inadequate in resisting rotational loads in cadaveric specimens.

Clinical study has further confirmed the importance of the PL bundle in the rotatory stability of the knee. With the use of high-speed in vivo steriography, Tashman and colleagues [23] detected that SB ACL reconstruction restored AP stability but failed to restore normal rotational knee kinematics with dynamic loading. The reconstructed knees were found to be more externally rotated than the contralateral native knees, leading to speculation that the abnormal joint motions detected may explain the high incidence of long-term joint degeneration and inconsistent ability to return to previous levels of activity after ACL reconstruction. Likewise, Georgoulis and colleagues [24] assessed tibial rotation in vivo after SB ACL reconstruction and found that although anteroposterior translation was restored, tibial rotation was not. Recently, a novel rotatory measurement system incorporating three-dimensional electromagnetic sensors enabled Yagi and colleagues [25] to reveal through the pivot-shift test that double-bundle (DB) ACL reconstruction is more rotationally stable than SB AM or PL reconstruction in 60 patients at 1-year follow-up. Similarly, in an evaluation of the pivot-shift test after ACL reconstruction with an optically based computer-assisted navigation system, Colombet and colleagues [26] demonstrated that SB AM reconstruction was inferior to SB PL reconstruction in restoration of rotational stability.

It can be concluded from both biomechanical and in vivo clinical research that the current SB ACL reconstructions succeed in stabilizing the knee, but they neither restore normal knee kinematics fully nor reproduce normal ligament function. The PL bundle plays a critical role in rotational stability of the knee, and current SB techniques serve primarily to restore only the AM bundle. To restore knee kinematics fully, it is necessary to restore both functional bundles of the ACL. For complete rupture of the ACL, DB reconstruction provides an anatomically based treatment approach [27] and is being used with promising results [4,28–34].

SURGICAL TECHNIQUE: ANATOMIC DOUBLE-BUNDLE ANTERIOR CRUCIATE LIGAMENT RECONSTRUCTION

The authors currently use a three-portal arthroscopic-assisted technique for DB ACL reconstruction that has evolved from previous published reports (Fig. 4) [27]. The technique is predicated on adequate visualization of the native anatomy. Diagnostic arthroscopy is performed with the knee in 90° of flexion, and the rupture pattern of the AM and PL bundles is determined. The authors routinely place the arthroscope in the AM portal, facilitating visualization of the femoral insertion of the ACL and virtually eliminating the need for notchplasty. In the case of complete rupture or stretching of both bundles, DB reconstruction is performed.

The femoral and tibial insertion sites are marked with a thermal device (Vulcan; Smith and Nephew, Andover, Massachusetts), and the midsubstance of the ligament remnants is resected. The peripheral attachments are preserved when possible to maintain the proprioceptive fibers that are present there [35,36]. When choosing tunnel position, the authors rely first on the soft tissue insertional anatomy, followed by the bony architecture, and finally on preconceived or accepted reference measurements or angles. Care is taken to preserve the superior border of the femoral AM insertion, because it serves as an important anatomic guide for anatomic tunnel placement (Figs. 5 and 6). The authors' typical graft choice for each bundle is a doubled-over tibialis anterior

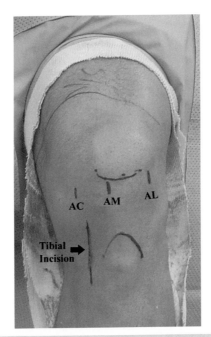

Fig. 4. Left knee: surgical incisions for ACL surgery: anterolateral portal (AL), anteromedial portal (AM), accessory medial portal (AC), and anteromedial tibial incision.

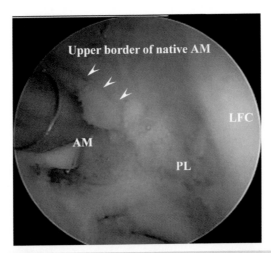

Fig. 5. Left knee: femoral ACL insertion. With the knee in 90° of flexion, the anteromedial (AM) and posterolateral (PL) bundle insertions are marked with a thermal device. Care is taken to preserve the superior border of the anteromedial bundle fibers, which serve as the upper limit for tunnel placement. LFC, lateral femoral condyle.

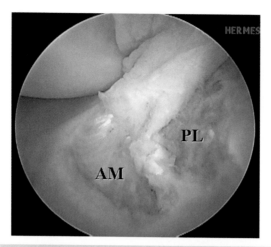

Fig. 6. Left knee: tibial ACL insertion. The oval anteromedial (AM) and circular posterolateral (PL) tibial insertions are marked with a thermal device.

allograft, although multiple graft options are available. Fixation typically is performed using an EndoButton (Smith and Nephew; Andover, Massachusetts) on the femoral side and a bioabsorbable screw on the tibial side, with or without staple augmentation.

The PL bundle femoral tunnel is drilled first, through an accessory medial portal, with a 6- or 7-mm diameter acorn reamer and the knee in hyperflexion. The center of the PL bundle insertion is approximately 5 to 7 mm posterior to and 3 mm superior to the border of the anterior articular cartilage (Fig. 7).

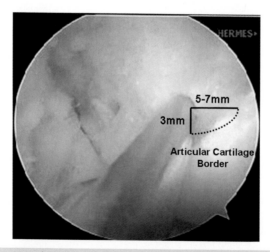

Fig. 7. Left knee: posterolateral tunnel. The center of the posterolateral bundle insertion is 5 to 7 mm posterior and 3 mm superior to the border of the anterior articular cartilage.

Once a depth of 20 mm is reached, the EndoButton drill (Smith and Nephew, Andover, Massachusetts) is advanced through the tunnel to cannulate the lateral femoral cortex for EndoButton passage. The tunnel is measured, and the depth is increased appropriately with a hand reamer to allow EndoButton passage and flipping.

Next, one tibial tunnel is drilled for each bundle. With a tip ACUFEX drill-guide (Smith and Nephew; Andover, Massachusetts) set at 45°, a guide pin is placed in the center of the T-shaped AM bundle tibial insertion site. Next, another guide pin is placed in the PL aspect of the tibial ACL insertion, approximately 3 to 5 mm from the posterior aspect of the triangle formed by the posterior cruciate ligament, the lateral meniscus posterior root, and the AM bundle insertion site (Fig. 8). The tibial tunnels subsequently are created over the guide wire to a diameter of 7 to 8 mm (AM) and 6 to 7 mm (PL), using a compaction drill and serial dilators (Figs. 9 and 10).

The femoral AM tunnel is created last. In many patients, a cruciate ridge of bone is present between the AM and PL bundles on the femoral insertion, facilitating identification of the correct AM tunnel position, which lies posterior to it (Fig. 11). In the authors' experience in placing this tunnel in the anatomic position, a transtibial approach through the AM tunnel is successful only about 50% of the time; in the other 50% of cases the tunnel is placed too high, above the superior border of the native AM bundle (Fig. 12). This erroneous placement can lead to posterior cruciate ligament impingement, vertical graft orientation, loss of knee flexion, and graft stretch-out. Drilling the AM femoral tunnel through the PL tibial tunnel improves accuracy to 70%, and the AM

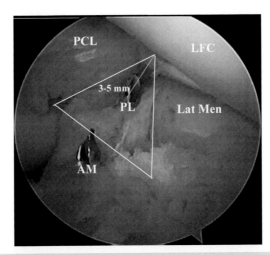

Fig. 8. Left knee: tunnel guide wires have been placed in the center of the anteromedial (AM) and posterolateral (PL) bundle tibial insertion sites. The center of the PL bundle is 3 to 5 mm from the posterior aspect of the triangle formed by the posterior cruciate ligament (PCL), lateral meniscus (Lat Men), posterior root, and anteromedial bundle insertion site. LFC, lateral femoral condyle.

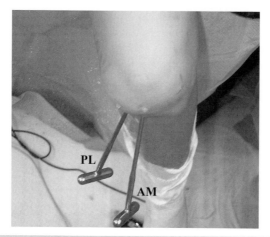

Fig. 9. Left knee: overhead photograph demonstrating orientation of anteromedial (AM) and posterolateral (PL) tibial tunnel dilators.

femoral tunnel can be placed correctly through the accessory medial portal in 99% of the cases (Fig. 13). The primary advantage of drilling transtibially for the AM femoral tunnel is the creation of a longer tunnel that diverges from the PL femoral tunnel, and the authors routinely attempt this approach first before using the accessory medial portal. Alternative methods for drilling the AM femoral tunnel include retrograde drilling, the use of a rear-entry drill guide, and flexible over-the-top drill guides that are based off of the posterior wall of the lateral femoral condyle.

Once all four tunnels are created, the PL graft is passed first, followed by the AM graft. Femoral fixation is performed, and the grafts are preconditioned

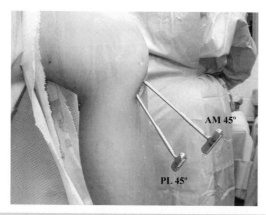

Fig. 10. Left knee: lateral photograph demonstrating orientation of anteromedial (AM) and posterolateral (PL) tibial tunnel dilators. The tibial guide is set at 45° for both tunnels.

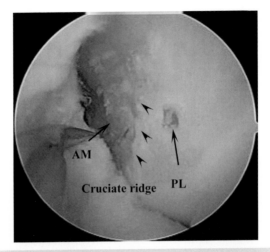

Fig. 11. Left knee: cruciate ridge on femoral insertion of ACL dividing the anteromedial (AM) and posterolateral (PL) bundle attachment sites.

with 25 cycles of maximum manual tension. The PL bundle is fixed to the tibia in full extension, and the AM bundle is fixed in 60° of knee flexion (Figs. 14–19). If the femoral tunnel is not long enough to allow use of an EndoButton, an EndoLoop (Smith and Nephew; Andover, Massachusetts) is used, and a 4.5-mm bicortical screw-post and washer is placed through the EndoLoop.

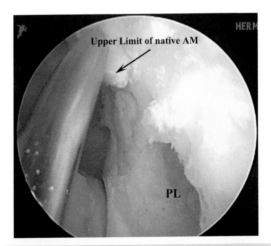

Fig. 12. Left knee: anteromedial femoral tunnel. Attempt at creating the anteromedial femoral tunnel through the anteromedial tibial tunnel. Guide wire placement using this approach will result in placement of the anteromedial graft superior to the upper limit of the native anteromedial bundle (AM). PL, posterolateral graft.

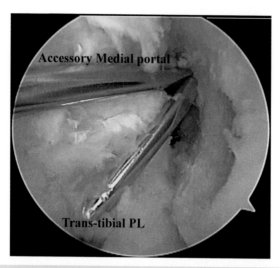

Fig. 13. Left knee: anteromedial femoral tunnel. Creation of the anteromedial femoral tunnel through either the accessory medial portal or tibial posterolateral tunnel (PL) results in anatomic placement of the anteromedial bundle.

SURGICAL TECHNIQUE: SINGLE-BUNDLE AUGMENTATION

Depending on the mechanism of injury, a partial tear of the ACL can occur, sparing either the AM or the PL bundle. Typically, isolated AM bundle tears present primarily with anteroposterior instability and increased laxity on Lachman examination, whereas isolated PL bundle tears present with

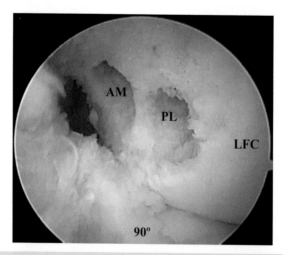

Fig. 14. Left knee: the anteromedial (AM) and posterolateral (PL) femoral tunnels have been created in the anatomic position. LFC, lateral femoral condyle.

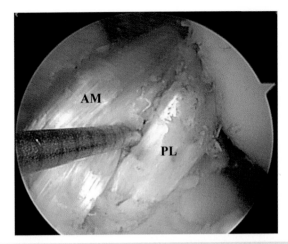

Fig. 15. Left knee: anteromedial (AM) bundle graft passage and fixation at 60° of knee flexion. The posterolateral (PL) bundle has been passed first and fixed in full extension.

rotatory instability and increased pivot-shift. Likewise, in failed SB ACL reconstruction, symptomatic rotatory instability and increased pivot-shift can occur because of the lack of a functioning PL bundle [37]. In all these instances SB augmentation can be performed. The AM or PL bundle graft is placed using the technique described for DB reconstruction, with the intact bundle preserved in situ.

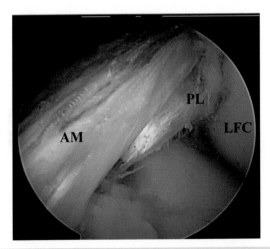

Fig. 16. Left knee: final result, anatomic double-bundle ACL reconstruction. AM, anteromedial; PL, posterolateral. LFC, lateral femoral condyle.

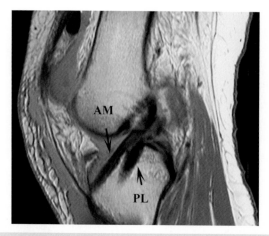

Fig. 17. Left knee: sagittal MRI, anatomic double-bundle ACL reconstruction. AM, anteromedial; PL, posterolateral.

CLINICAL RESULTS: DOUBLE-BUNDLE RECONSTRUCTION

From November 2003 to January 2007, the senior author (FHF) has performed 388 anatomical DB ACL reconstructions. Of 312 primary cases, 295 patients (95%) had primary DB reconstruction, and 16 patients (5%) had primary SB augmentation. Of 76 revision cases, 52 patients (68%) had DB reconstruction, and 24 patients (32%) had secondary SB augmentation.

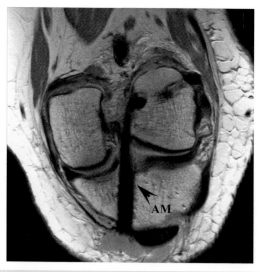

Fig. 18. Left knee: oblique coronal MRI, anteromedial bundle (AM) of the anatomic double-bundle ACL reconstruction.

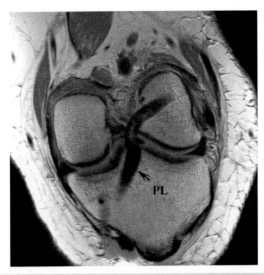

Fig. 19. Left knee: oblique coronal MRI, posterolateral bundle (PL) of the anatomic double-bundle ACL reconstruction.

A prospective study was designed to evaluate the clinical outcomes of these patients. Outcome measurements included the Lachman test, pivot-shift test, KT-2000, range of motion, and overall International Knee Documentation Committee (IKDC) rating. Short-term results show that the range of motion after primary DB ACL reconstruction is better than after primary SB ACL reconstruction at 1, 4, and 12 weeks postoperatively following the same rehabilitation protocol (F.H. Fu, unpublished data, 2007). These patients are being followed continuously to determine additional long-term advantages of DB reconstruction over SB reconstruction. At this time, the initial 100 consecutive patients who underwent primary DB ACL reconstruction have been followed for an average of approximately 2 years. Clinical examinations suggest that DB ACL reconstruction effectively restores anteroposterior stability. Approximately 94% of patients had excellent or good IKDC ratings. In the initial 100 patients there were 4 failures, 3 of which required DB revision surgery. For the augmentation and DB revision cases, preliminary results are being reviewed and seem promising. Further study is warranted and is ongoing.

GRAFT CHOICE: DOUBLE-BUNDLE RECONSTRUCTION

In 1999, the majority of members of the American Orthopaedic Society of Sports Medicine reported bone-patellar tendon-bone (BPTB) autograft as the graft of choice for ACL reconstruction [38]. Although considered the gold standard, the graft has drawbacks. The most commonly reported problems result from harvest morbidity, including anterior knee pain [39–45], pain with kneeling [45–48], patellar tendon rupture [49], patellar tendonitis [40,50], patellar fracture [51], alteration of quadriceps function [39,48,52], loss of terminal extension [39,44,53], and numbness or dysesthesias caused by cutting the infrapatellar branch of the saphenous nerve [46]. Additionally, a higher rate of osteoarthritis has been seen on radiographs following ACL reconstruction with BPTB than with hamstring tendons (HT) [45,54,55]. As an alternative, HT grafts have been selected because of increased strength [56,57], improved cosmesis, and lower graft-site morbidity [58,59]. Reduced peak torque of the hamstring muscles has been reported [50,60,61], however, and concern exists over a tendency toward residual laxity and tunnel widening after reconstruction [46,62–65]. Achilles tendon allograft provides a bone block with a strong tendinous attachment and is used by some for ACL reconstruction. Quadriceps tendon-bone (QTB) autograft and allograft are used also, although less commonly.

Ideally, the mechanical strength of the graft choice will be equal or superior to the injured ACL. Woo and colleagues [56] found the native ACL to have an ultimate load to failure of 2160 Newton (N) when specimens from persons 22 to 35 years of age were tested in the anatomic position. The 10-mm QTB graft has been found to have an ultimate tensile load of 2352 N [66,67]. Patellar tendon autograft has been found to have a maximum tensile strength of 2977 N [68]. In comparison, quadrupled HT has been found have a higher ultimate tensile strength of 4108 N, suggesting a potential relative benefit in using this graft source for ACL reconstruction [57]. The HT graft is the stiffest (776 N/mm), followed by BPTB (620 N/mm), QTB (463 N/mm), and the native ACL (242 N/mm). The QTB graft is the largest (62 mm^2), followed by HT (53 mm^2), the native ACL (44 mm^2), and BPTB (35 mm^2). Despite differing mechanical profiles, numerous clinical studies have concluded that there are no significant functional differences between the two most common graft choices, quadrupled HT and BPTB, for ACL reconstruction [15,44,47,48,53–55,69,70].

Achilles tendon allografts allow bone-to-bone healing on one end of the graft and typically tendon-to-bone healing on the other. Recently, Gasser and Uppal [71] have described suturing a free bone block to the tendinous end of an Achilles autograft, thereby allowing bone-to-bone healing on the tibia as well as the femur; preliminary results on 40 patients show no failures of fixation.

The use of full-thickness central-third QTB graft was popularized by Blauth [72] and Fulkerson [73]. Potential advantages of the use of QTB instead of BPTB include preservation of the infrapatellar branch of the saphenous nerve, avoidance of infrapatellar scarring and patella baja from violation of the patellar tendon, and improved isokinetic recovery of thigh strength [74]. Like the BPTB graft, the QTB provides the option for bone-to-bone healing at one point of fixation. At an average of 62 months' follow-up, Chen and colleagues [75] reported the results of SB ACL reconstruction with autogenous QTB in 34 patients: 82% of patients had less than 2 mm of residual laxity, and 94% achieved good or excellent results by Lysholm knee rating. In a similar study, Lee and colleagues [76] reported mean residual laxity of 2 mm and a Lysholm score of

90 in 67 patients who underwent SB ACL reconstruction with QTB at mean follow-up of 41 months; at 2 years extension peak torque was restored to the contralateral knee in 89% of patients. A surgical technique for SB ACL reconstruction with quadriceps tendon autograft, without a bone block, using bioabsorbable cross-pin fixation also has been described, without clinical follow-up [77]. Recently, Kim and colleagues [78] have described a surgical technique for a modified DB ACL reconstruction with QTB, in which the patellar bone block is secured in one tibial tunnel, and the graft is split into two strands that are placed into two femoral tunnels.

The use of allograft in ACL reconstruction benefits the patient most significantly by avoiding morbidity at the autograft harvest site and allowing more expeditious recovery from surgery [79,80]. Given the significant amount of tissue required to perform an anatomic, four-tunnel DB ACL reconstruction, it is likely that allograft will remain invaluable in the surgical technique until further advances in tissue engineering occur. Potential concerns regarding allograft use include disease transmission [81–83], bacterial infection [84,85], slower incorporation [86], immunologic reactions, effects from processing [87–90], and cost. Common graft options include tibialis anterior, posterior tibialis, Achilles, BPTB, QTB, and HT.

Before the use of polymerase chain reaction testing, the HIV transmission rate from allograft was estimated to be less than 1 in 1.7 million; the rate should be lower with the implementation of more sensitive testing technology [81,82]. In 2001, the American Association of Tissue Banks reported that in the prior 5 years more than 2 million musculoskeletal allografts were used with no documented incident of viral infectious disease transmission caused by an allograft [91]. In 2006, approximately 1.5 million bone and tissue allografts were implanted, most of which were bone-tendon-bone grafts [92].

Despite the cost of allograft tendon, in a cost analysis of 122 patients undergoing ACL reconstruction with either BPTB autograft or freeze-dried Achilles tendon allograft, Cole and colleagues [93] found the use of autograft to be more expensive, primarily because increased operating room time and the greater likelihood of overnight hospitalization for autograft procedures offset the cost of the allograft itself. Multiple studies have compared the use of allograft with autograft for ACL reconstruction and have found no differences in long-term follow-up, suggesting that other factors probably play a more significant role in determining surgical success [94–96].

THE FUTURE

To fulfill the demand of tissue for ACL grafts and in hopes of addressing the drawbacks of autograft and allograft, synthetic graft materials have been studied for ACL implantation since the early 1970s. This research has taken on added significance with the advent of DB ACL reconstruction, which uses more tissue than standard SB reconstruction. Although early synthetic grafts provided satisfactory initial strength because of the stiff materials used in their composition, they were associated with concerning complications including foreign-body inflammation, synovitis, and graft rupture [97–100]. These clinical failures stimulated interest in tissue engineering as a safe, alternative source for graft tissue.

The research involving tissue-engineered ACL grafts focuses on the three essential components: (1) cells that are capable of proliferation and matrix synthesis, (2) biodegradable scaffolds that facilitate cell growth, and (3) an environment that provides nutrient and appropriate regulatory stimuli. Fibroblasts from various mesenchymal tissues have been shown to proliferate, synthesize collagen, and respond to mechanical and biochemical growth factors [101–103]. Bone marrow stem cells (BMSC), because of their differentiation potential, also were tested as candidates for the cell source of tissue-engineered ACL graft. A comparative evaluation of goat BMSCs, ACL fibroblasts, and skin fibroblasts was undertaken to evaluate the optimal cell source for ACL engineering. After being seeded onto a degradable suture material for a maximum of 12 days, BMSCs showed the highest DNA content and collagen production, although each of the cell types attached, proliferated, and synthesized extracellular matrix rich in collagen type I [104].

The scaffold is another elemental component in the tissue-engineered ACL graft. Of the materials studied, collagen received a great deal of early interest. Dunn and colleagues [101] and Bellincampi and colleagues [102] observed fibroblast proliferation on bovine collagen both in vitro and in vivo. The use of collagen scaffold was limited, however, because tissue ingrowth in these scaffolds was inconsistent, and the implants failed to regain a mechanical strength comparable to that of the native ligament. Silk scaffold has shown promise as an alternative in ligament replacement. "Wire-rope" scaffold, composed of bundles of fibers wound into fibrils that then are woven into cords, shows mechanical properties comparable to the native ACL [105–107]. Seeded with human BMSCs and subjected to cyclic translational and rotational strain, the silk scaffolds can induce collagen synthesis and cell differentiation [105,106]. Cell attachment and proliferation were improved further by modification of this matrix with short polypeptide sequences, such as arginine-glycine-aspartic acid [108].

Synthetic materials are potentially useful for ACL tissue engineering. Laurencin and colleagues have developed a three-dimensional braided poly (lactic-co-glycolic acid) (PLGA) scaffold for ACL tissue engineering [109]. More recently, three-dimensional braided scaffolds composed of poly L-lactic acid and precoated with fibronectin seems to enable better cell proliferation and long-term mechanical properties than obtained with PLGA [110]. In addition, the ACL, medial collateral ligament, Achilles tendon, and patellar tendon have been studied as potential cell sources for a tissue-engineered ACL [111]. Biologic materials such as hyaluronic acid, chitosan, and alginate are potential candidates for ACL scaffolds, because they are inherently biocompatible and provide good cell adhesion. Modified hyaluronic acid–based scaffolds and alginate-chitosan hybrid polymers were shown to be good substrates for cell growth and collagen type I expression [112,113].

Appropriate regulatory stimuli, including mechanical and biologic stimuli, are important in the development of tissue-engineered ACL grafts. Fibroblasts within ligaments frequently are exposed to dynamic stress, and mechanical stimuli are indispensable in maintaining ligament strength. Berry and colleagues [114] found cell alignment and cellular metabolism were dependent on the applied strain profile, as well as on cell proliferation, collagen synthesis, and matrix metalloproteinase production [115]. To improve cell proliferation and matrix production, many growth factors have been used in ACL tissue engineering [116]. Future studies should focus on the working mechanism, temporal demand, sustainable release, and physiologic concentration of these growth factors. Eventually it is anticipated that a graft will be engineered with a biologic and mechanical profile analogous to the native ACL, providing a successful substrate for ACL reconstruction.

References

[1] Griffin LY, Agel J, Albolm MJ, et al. Noncontact anterior cruciate ligament injuries: risk factors and prevention strategies. J Am Acad Orthop Surg 2000;8(3):141–50.

[2] O'Rahilly R. The early prenatal development of the human knee joint. J Anat 1951;85: 166–70.

[3] Gardner E, O'Rahilly R. The early development of the knee joint in staged human embryos. J Anat 1968;102:289–99.

[4] Chhabra A, Starman JS, Ferretti M, et al. Anatomic, radiographic, biomechanical, and kinematic evaluation of the anterior cruciate ligament and its two functional bundles. J Bone Joint Surg Am 2006;88(Suppl 4):2–10.

[5] Girgis FG, Marshal JL, Monajem A. The cruciate ligaments of the knee joint. Anatomical, functional and experimental analysis. Clin Orthop Relat Res 1975;106:216–31.

[6] Amis AA, Dawkins GP. Functional anatomy of the anterior cruciate ligament. Fibre bundle actions related to ligament replacements and injuries. J Bone Joint Surg Br 1991;73(2): 260–7.

[7] Harner CD, Baek GH, Vogrin TM, et al. Quantitative analysis of human cruciate ligament insertions. Arthroscopy 1999;15(7):741–9.

[8] Odensten M, Gillquist J. Functional anatomy of the anterior cruciate ligament and a rationale for reconstruction. J Bone Joint Surg Am 1985;67:257–62.

[9] Takahashi M, Doi M, Abe M, et al. Anatomical study of the femoral and tibial insertions of the anteromedial and posterolateral bundles of human anterior cruciate ligament. Am J Sports Med 2006;34:787–92.

[10] Duthon VB, Barea C, Abrassart S, et al. Anatomy of the anterior cruciate ligament. Knee Surg Sports Traumatol Arthrosc 2006;14:204–13.

[11] Mochizuki T, Muneta T, Nagase T, et al. Cadaveric knee observation study for describing anatomic femoral tunnel placement for two-bundle anterior cruciate ligament reconstruction. Arthroscopy 2006;22(4):356–61.

[12] Freedman KB, D'Amato MJ, Nedeff DD, et al. Arthroscopic anterior cruciate ligament reconstruction: a metaanalysis comparing patellar tendon and hamstring tendon autografts. Am J Sports Med 2003;31:2–11.

[13] Yunes M, Richmond JC, Engels EA, et al. Patellar versus hamstring tendons in anterior cruciate ligament reconstruction: a meta-analysis. Arthroscopy 2001;17:248–57.

[14] Anderson AF, Snyder RB, Lipscomb AB Jr. Anterior cruciate ligament reconstruction. A prospective randomized study of three surgical methods. Am J Sports Med 2001;29:272–9.

[15] Aune AK, Holm I, Risberg MA, et al. Four-strand hamstring tendon autograft compared with patellar tendon-bone autograft for anterior cruciate ligament reconstruction. A randomized study with two-year follow-up. Am J Sports Med 2001;29:722–8.

[16] Fithian DC, Paxton EW, Stone ML, et al. Prospective trial of a treatment algorithm for the management of the anterior cruciate ligament-injured knee. Am J Sports Med 2005;33(3): 333–4.

[17] Kocher MS, Steadman JR, Briggs KK, et al. Relationships between objective assessment of ligament stability and subjective assessment of symptoms and function after anterior cruciate ligament reconstruction. Am J Sports Med 2004;32:629–34.

[18] Sakane M, Fox RJ, Woo SL. In situ forces in the anterior cruciate ligament and its bundles in response to anterior tibial loads. J Orthop Res 1997;15(2):285–93.

[19] Gabriel MT, Wong EK, Wool SL, et al. Distribution of in situ forces in the anterior cruciate ligament in response to rotatory loads. J Orthop Res 2004;22(1):85–9.

[20] Zantop T, Herbort M, Raschke MJ, et al. The role of the anteromedial and posterolateral bundles of the anterior cruciate ligament in anterior tibial translation and internal rotation. Am J Sports Med 2007;35:223–7.

[21] Woo SL, Kanamori A, Zeminski J, et al. The effectiveness of reconstruction of the anterior cruciate ligament with hamstrings and patellar tendon. A cadaveric study comparing anterior tibial and rotational loads. J Bone Joint Surg Am 2002;84:907–14.

[22] Yagi M, Wong EK, Kanamori A, et al. Biomechanical analysis of an anatomic anterior cruciate ligament reconstruction. Am J Sports Med 2002;30:660–6.

[23] Tashman S, Collon D, Anderson K, et al. Abnormal rotational knee motion during running after anterior cruciate ligament reconstruction. Am J Sports Med 2004;32: 975–83.

[24] Georgoulis AD, Ristanis S, Chouliaras V, et al. Tibial rotation is not restored after ACL reconstruction with a hamstring graft. Clin Orthop Relat Res 2007;454:89–94.

[25] Yagi M, Ryosuke K, Nagamune K, et al. Double-bundle ACL reconstruction can improve rotational stability. Clin Orthop Relat Res 2007;454:100–7.

[26] Colombet P, Robinson J, Christel P, et al. Using navigation to measure rotation kinematics during ACL reconstruction. Clin Orthop Relat Res 2007;454:59–65.

[27] Vidal AF, Brucker PU, Fu FH, et al. Anatomic double-bundle anterior cruciate ligament reconstruction using tibialis anterior tendon autografts. Operative Techniques in Orthopaedics 2005;15:140–5.

[28] Hara K, Kubo T, Suginoshita T, et al. Reconstruction of the anterior cruciate ligament using a double bundle. Arthroscopy 2000;16:860–4.

[29] Muneta T, Sekiya I, Yagishita K, et al. Two-bundle reconstruction of the anterior cruciate ligament using semitendinosus tendon with EndoButtons: operative technique and preliminary results. Arthroscopy 1999;15(6):618–24.

[30] Hamada M, Shino K, Horibe S, et al. Single-versus bi-socket anterior cruciate ligament reconstruction using autogenous multiple-stranded hamstring tendons with EndoButton femoral fixation: a prospective study. Arthroscopy 2001;17(8):801–7.

[31] Colombet P, Robinson J, Jambou S, et al. Two-bundle, four-tunnel anterior cruciate ligament reconstruction. Knee Surg Sports Traumatol Arthrosc 2006;14:629–36.

[32] Marcacci M, Molgora AP, Zaffagnini S, et al. Anatomic double-bundle anterior cruciate ligament reconstruction with hamstrings. Arthroscopy 2003;19:540–6.

[33] Takeuchi R, Saito T, Mituhashi S, et al. Double-bundle anatomic anterior cruciate ligament reconstruction using bone-hamstring-bone composite graft. Arthroscopy 2002;18: 550–5.

[34] Yasuda K, Kondo E, Ichiyama H, et al. Anatomic reconstruction of the anteromedial and posterolateral bundles of the anterior cruciate ligament using hamstring tendon grafts. Arthroscopy 2004;20:1015–25.

[35] Kennedy JC, Alexander IJ, Hayes KC. Nerve supply of the human knee and its functional importance. Am J Sports Med 1982;10:329–35.

[36] Schutte MJ, Dabezies EJ, Zimny ML, et al. Neural anatomy of the human anterior cruciate ligament. J Bone Joint Surg Am 1987;69:243–7.

[37] Brucker PU, Zelle BA, Fu FH. Revision after anterior cruciate ligament reconstruction by restoration of the posterolateral bundle. Operative Techniques in Orthopaedics 2005; 15:146–50.

[38] Delay BS, Smolinski RJ, Wind WM, et al. Current practices and opinions in ACL reconstruction and rehabilitation: results of a survey of the American Orthopaedic Society for Sports Medicine. Am J Knee Surg 2001;14:85–91.

[39] Sachs RA, Daniel DM, Stone ML, et al. Patellofemoral problems after anterior cruciate ligament reconstruction. Am J Sports Med 1989;17(6):760–5.

[40] Aglietti P, Buzzi R, D'Andria S, et al. Patellofemoral problems after intraarticular anterior cruciate ligament reconstruction. Clin Orthop Relat Res 1993;288:195–204.

[41] Cory IS, Webb JM, Clingeleffer AJ, et al. Arthroscopic reconstruction of the anterior cruciate ligament: a comparison of patellar tendon autograft and four-strand hamstring tendon autograft. Am J Sports Med 1999;27:444–54.

[42] Bach BR Jr, Tradonsky S, Bojchuk J, et al. Arthroscopically assisted anterior cruciate ligament reconstruction using patellar tendon autograft: five-to nine-year follow-up evaluation. Am J Sports Med 1998;26:20–9.

[43] Kleipool AE, van Loon T, Marti RK. Pain after use of the central third of the patellar tendon for cruciate ligament reconstruction. 33 patients followed 2-3 years. Acta Orthop Scand 1994;65:62–6.

[44] Shaieb MD, Kan DM, Chang SK, et al. A prospective randomized comparison of patellar tendon versus semitendinosus and gracilis tendon autografts for anterior cruciate ligament reconstruction. Am J Sports Med 2002;30(2):214–20.

[45] Pinczewski LA, Lyman J, Salmon LJ, et al. A 10-year comparison of anterior cruciate ligament reconstruction with hamstring tendon and patellar tendon autograft: a controlled, prospective trial. Am J Sports Med 2007; [e-pub doi:10.1177/0363546506296042].

[46] Aglietti P, Giron F, Buzzi R, et al. Anterior cruciate ligament reconstruction: bone-patellar tendon-bone compared with double semitendinosus and gracilis tendon grafts. A prospective, randomized clinical trial. J Bone Joint Surg 2004;86:2143–55.

[47] Ejerhed L, Kartus J, Senert N, et al. Patellar tendon or semitendinosus tendon autografts for anterior cruciate ligament reconstruction? A prospective randomized study with a two-year follow-up. Am J Sports Med 2003;31:19–25.

[48] Feller JA, Webster KE. A randomized comparison of patellar tendon and hamstring tendon anterior cruciate ligament reconstruction. Am J Sports Med 2003;31:564–73.

[49] Marumoto JM, Mitsunaga MM, Richardson AB, et al. Late patellar tendon ruptures after removal of the central third for anterior cruciate ligament reconstruction. A report of two cases. Am J Sports Med 1996;24:698–701.

[50] Marder RA, Raskind JR, Carroll M. Prospective evaluation of arthroscopically assisted anterior cruciate ligament reconstruction. Patellar tendon versus semitendinosus and gracilis tendons. Am J Sports Med 1991;19(5):478–84.

[51] Simonian PT, Mann FA, Mandt PR. Indirect forces and patella fracture after anterior cruciate ligament reconstruction with the patellar ligament. Case report. Am J Knee Surg 1995;8:60–5.

[52] Rosenberg TD, Franklin JL, Baldwin GN, et al. Extensor mechanism function after patellar tendon graft harvest for anterior cruciate ligament reconstruction. Am J Sports Med 1992;20(5):519–26.

[53] Eriksson K, Anderberg P, Hamberg P, et al. A comparison of quadruple semitendinosus and patellar tendon grafts in reconstruction of the anterior cruciate ligament. J Bone Joint Surg Br 2001;83(3):348–54.

[54] Sajovic M, Vengust V, Komadina R, et al. A prospective, randomized comparison of semitendinosus and gracilis tendon versus patellar tendon autografts for anterior cruciate ligament reconstruction: five-year follow-up. Am J Sports Med 2006;34(12): 1933–40.

[55] Roe J, Pinczewski LA, Russell VJ, et al. A 7-year follow-up of patellar tendon and hamstring tendon grafts for arthroscopic anterior cruciate ligament reconstruction. Am J Sports Med 2006;33:1337–45.

[56] Woo SL, Hollis JM, Adams DJ, et al. Tensile properties of the human femur-anterior cruciate ligament-tibia complex. The effects of specimen age and orientation. Am J Sports Med 1991;19:217–25.

[57] Brown CH Jr, Steiner ME, Carson EW. The use of hamstring tendons for anterior cruciate ligament reconstruction. Technique and results. Clin Sports Med 1993;12:723–56.

[58] Cross MJ, Roger G, Kujawa P, et al. Regeneration of the semitendinosus and gracilis tendons following their transection for repair of the anterior cruciate ligament. Am J Sports Med 1992;20(2):221–3.

[59] Yasuda K, Tsujino J, Ohkoshi Y, et al. Graft site morbidity with autogenous semitendinosus and gracilis tendons. Am J Sports Med 1995;23:706–14.

[60] Nakamura N, Horibe S, Sasaki S, et al. Evaluation of active knee flexion and hamstring strength after anterior cruciate ligament reconstruction using hamstring tendons. Arthroscopy 2002;18(6):598–602.

[61] Adachi N, Ochi M, Uchio Y, et al. Harvesting hamstring tendons for ACL reconstruction influences postoperative hamstring muscle performance. Arch Orthop Trauma Surg 2003;123(9):460–5.

[62] Clatworthy MG, Annear P, Bulow JU, et al. Tunnel widening in anterior cruciate ligament reconstruction: a prospective evaluation of hamstring and patella tendon grafts. Knee Surg Sports Traumatol Arthrosc 1999;7(3):138–45.

[63] Aglietti P, Buzzi R, Zaccherotti G, et al. Patellar tendon versus doubled semitendinosus and gracilis tendons for anterior cruciate ligament reconstruction. Am J Sports Med 1994;22(2):211–8.

[64] Otero AL, Hutcheson L. A comparison of the doubled semitendinosus/gracilis and central third of the patellar tendon autografts in arthroscopic anterior cruciate ligament reconstruction. Arthroscopy 1993;9(2):143–8.

[65] Salmon LJ, Refshauge KM, Russell VJ, et al. Gender differences in outcome after anterior cruciate ligament reconstruction with hamstring tendon autograft. Am J Sports Med 2006;34:621–9.

[66] Staubli HU, Schatzmann L, Brunner P, et al. Mechanical tensile properties of the quadriceps tendon and patellar ligament in young adults. Am J Sports Med 1999;27(1):27–34.

[67] Harris NL, Smith DA, Lamoreaux L, et al. Central quadriceps tendon for anterior cruciate ligament reconstruction. Part I: morphometric and biomechanical evaluation. Am J Sports Med 1997;25(1):23–8.

[68] Noyes FR, Butler DL, Grood ES, et al. Biomechanical analysis of human ligament grafts used in knee-ligament repairs and reconstructions. J Bone Joint Surg Am 1984;66(3):344–52.

[69] Jansson KA, Linko E, Sandelin J, et al. A prospective randomized study of patellar versus hamstring tendon autografts for anterior cruciate ligament reconstruction. Am J Sports Med 2003;31:12–8.

[70] Laxdal G, Sernert N, Ejerhed L, et al. A prospective comparison of bone-patellar tendon-bone and hamstring tendon grafts for anterior cruciate ligament reconstruction in male patients. Knee Surg Sports Traumatol Arthrosc 2007;15(2):115–25.

[71] Gasser S, Uppal R. Anterior cruciate ligament reconstruction: a new technique for Achilles tendon preparation. Arthroscopy 2006;22(12):1365, e1–3.

[72] Blauth W. 2-strip substitution-plasty of the anterior cruciate ligament with the quadriceps tendon. Unfallheilkunde 1984;87:45–51.

[73] Fulkerson JP, Langeland R. An alternative cruciate reconstruction graft: the central quadriceps tendon. Arthroscopy 1995;11:252–4.

[74] Pigozzi F, Di Salvo V, Parisi A, et al. Isokinetic evaluation of anterior cruciate ligament reconstruction: quadriceps tendon versus patellar tendon. J Sports Med Phys Fitness 2004;44(3):288–93.

[75] Chen CH, Chuang TY, Wang KC, et al. Arthroscopic anterior cruciate ligament reconstruction with quadriceps tendon autograft: clinical outcome in 4-7 years. Knee Surg Sports Traumatol Arthrosc 2006;14(11):1077–85.

[76] Lee S, Seong SC, Jo H, et al. Outcome of anterior cruciate ligament reconstruction using quadriceps tendon autograft. Arthroscopy 2004;20(8):795–802.

[77] Antonogiannakis E, Yiannakopoulos CK, Hiotis I, et al. Arthroscopic anterior cruciate ligament reconstruction using quadriceps tendon autograft and bioabsorbable cross-pin fixation. Arthroscopy 2005;21(7):894.

[78] Kim SJ, Jung KA, Song DH. Arthroscopic double-bundle anterior cruciate ligament reconstruction using autogenous quadriceps tendon. Arthroscopy 2006;22(7):797, e1–5.

[79] West RV, Harner CD. Graft selection in anterior cruciate ligament reconstruction. J Am Acad Orthop Surg 2005;13(3):197–207.

[80] Miller MD, Harner CD. The use of allograft. Techniques and results. Clin Sports Med 1993;12(4):757–70.

[81] Buck BE, Malinin TI, Brown MD. Bone transplantation and human immunodeficiency virus. An estimate of risk of acquired immunodeficiency syndrome (AIDS). Clin Orthop Relat Res 1989;240:129–36.

[82] Busch MP, Lee LL, Satten GA, et al. Time course of detection of viral and serologic marker preceding human immunodeficiency virus type 1 seroconversion: implications for screening of blood and tissue donors. Transfusion 1995;35:91–7.

[83] Centers for Disease Control and Prevention (CDC). Hepatitis C virus transmission from an antibody-negative organ and tissue donor—United States, 2000–2002. MMWR Morb Mortal Wkly Rep 2003;52:273–6.

[84] Centers for Disease Control and Prevention (CDC). Update: allograft-associated bacterial infections. MMWR Morb Mortal Wkly Rep 2002;51:207–10.

[85] Centers for Disease Control (CDC). Invasive Streptococcus pyogenes after allograft implantation—Colorado, 2003. MMWR Morb Mortal Wkly Rep 2003;52:1173–6.

[86] Jackson DW, Corsetti J, Simon TM. Biologic incorporation of allograft anterior cruciate ligament replacements. Clin Orthop Relat Res 1996;324:126–33.

[87] Wilson TC, Kantaras A, Atay A, et al. Tunnel enlargement after anterior cruciate ligament surgery. Am J Sports Med 2004;32:543–9.

[88] Gibbons MJ, Butler DL, Grood ES, et al. Effects of gamma irradiation on the initial mechanical and material properties of goat bone-patellar tendon-bone allografts. J Orthop Res 1991;9:209–18.

[89] Godette GA, Kopta JA, Egle DM. Biomechanical effects of gamma irradiation on fresh frozen allografts in vivo. Orthopedics 1996;19:649–53.

[90] Vangsness CT Jr, Wagner PP, Moore TM, et al. Overview of safety issues concerning the preparation and processing of soft-tissue allografts. Arthroscopy 2006;22(12):1351–8.

[91] Woll JE. Standards for tissue banking. McLean (VA): American Association of Tissue Banks; 2001.

[92] Centers for Disease Control and Prevention. About tissue transplants. March 20, 2006. Available at: http://www.cdc.gov/ncidod/dhqp/tissueTransplantsFAQ.html. Accessed January 28, 2007.

[93] Cole DW, Ginn TA, Chen GJ, et al. Cost comparison of anterior cruciate ligament reconstruction: autograft versus allograft. Arthroscopy 2005;21(7):786–90.

[94] Poehling GG, Curl WW, Lee CA, et al. Analysis of outcomes of anterior cruciate ligament repair with 5-year follow-up: allograft versus autograft. Arthroscopy 2005;21(7):774–85.

[95] Kleipool AE, Zijl JA, Willems WJ. Arthroscopic anterior cruciate ligament reconstruction with bone-patellar tendon-bone allograft or autograft. A prospective study with an average follow up of 4 years. Knee Surg Sports Traumatol Arthrosc 1998;6(4):224–30.

[96] Shelton WR, Papendick L, Dukes AD. Autograft versus allograft anterior cruciate ligament reconstruction. Arthroscopy 1997;13(4):446–9.

[97] Guidoin MF, Marois Y, Bejui J, et al. Analysis of retrieved polymer fiber based replacements for the ACL. Biomaterials 2000;21(23):2461–74.

[98] Richmond JC, Manseau CJ, Patz R, et al. Anterior cruciate reconstruction using a Dacron ligament prosthesis. A long-term study. Am J Sports Med 1992;20(1):24–8.

[99] Bolton CW, Bruchman WC. The GORE-TEX expanded polytetrafluoroethylene prosthetic ligament. An in vitro and in vivo evaluation. Clin Orthop Relat Res 1985;196:202–13.

[100] Mody BA, Howard L, Harding ML, et al. The ABC carbon and polyester prosthetic ligament for ACL-deficient knees. Early results in 31 cases. J Bone Joint Surg Br 1993;75(5): 818–21.

[101] Dunn MG, Liesch JB, Tiku ML, et al. Development of fibroblast-seeded ligament analogs for ACL reconstruction. J Biomed Mater Res 1995;29(11):1363–71.

[102] Bellincampi LD, Closkey RF, Prasad R, et al. Viability of fibroblast-seeded ligament analogs after autogenous implantation. J Orthop Res 1998;16(4):414–20.

[103] Lin VS, Lee MC, O'Neal S, et al. Ligament tissue engineering using synthetic biodegradable fiber scaffolds. Tissue Eng 1999;5(5):443–52.

[104] Van Eijk F, Saris DB, Riesle J, et al. Tissue engineering of ligaments: a comparison of bone marrow stromal cells, anterior cruciate ligament, and skin fibroblasts as cell source. Tissue Eng 2004;10(5–6):893–903.

[105] Vunjak-Novakovic G, Altman G, Horan R. Tissue engineering of ligaments. Annu Rev Biomed Eng 2004;6:131–56.

[106] Altman GH, Horan RL, Martin I, et al. Cell differentiation by mechanical stress. FASEB J 2002;16(2):270–2.

[107] Altman GH, Horan RL, Lu HH, et al. Silk matrix for tissue engineered anterior cruciate ligaments. Biomaterials 2002;23(20):4131–41.

[108] Chen J, Altman GH, Karageorgiou V, et al. Human bone marrow stromal cell and ligament fibroblast responses on RGD-modified silk fibers. J Biomed Mater Res 2003;67(2): 559–70.

[109] Cooper JA, Lu HH, Ko FK, et al. Fiber-based tissue-engineered scaffold for ligament replacement: design considerations and in vitro evaluation. Biomaterials 2005;26(13): 1523–32.

[110] Lu HH, Cooper JA Jr, Manuel S, et al. Anterior cruciate ligament regeneration using braided biodegradable scaffolds: in vitro optimization studies. Biomaterials 2005;26(23): 4805–16.

[111] Cooper JA Jr, Bailey LO, Carter JN, et al. Evaluation of the anterior cruciate ligament, medial collateral ligament, Achilles tendon and patellar tendon as cell sources for tissue-engineered ligament. Biomaterials 2006;27(13):2747–54.

[112] Majima T, Funakosi T, Iwasaki N, et al. Alginate and chitosan polyion complex hybrid fibers for scaffolds in ligament and tendon tissue engineering. J Orthop Sci 2005;10(3): 302–7.

[113] Cristino S, Grassi F, Toneguzzi S, et al. Analysis of mesenchymal stem cells grown on a three-dimensional HYAFF 11-based prototype ligament scaffold. J Biomed Mater Res 2005;73(3):275–83.

[114] Berry CC, Cacou C, Lee DA, et al. Dermal fibroblasts respond to mechanical conditioning in a strain profile dependent manner. Biorheology 2003;40(1–3):337–45.

[115] Berry CC, Shelton JC, Bader DL, et al. Influence of external uniaxial cyclic strain on oriented fibroblast-seeded collagen gels. Tissue Eng 2003;9(4):613–24.

[116] Goh JC, Ouyang HW, Teoh SH, et al. Tissue-engineering approach to the repair and regeneration of tendons and ligaments. Tissue Eng 2003;9(Suppl 1):S31–44.

Clin Sports Med 26 (2007) 661–681

CLINICS IN SPORTS MEDICINE

ELSEVIER
SAUNDERS

Clinical Outcomes of Allograft Versus Autograft in Anterior Cruciate Ligament Reconstruction

Geoffrey S. Baer, MD, PhD[a], Christopher D. Harner, MD[a,b],*

[a]Department of Orthopaedic Surgery, University of Pittsburgh Medical Center, UPMC Center for Sports Medicine, 3200 S. Water Street, Pittsburgh, PA 15203, USA
[b]Center for Sports Medicine, University of Pittsburgh Medical Center, 3200 S. Water Street, Pittsburgh, PA 15203, USA

Anterior cruciate ligament (ACL) injuries are the most common complete ligamentous injury to the knee [1]. They occur mainly in the young athletic population, especially in young female athletes [2–4]. ACL injuries have been reported to occur in an estimated 1 in 3000 people in the United States population each year [5–8], with more than 100,000 ACL reconstructions performed annually [9–12]. Although bone-patellar tendon-bone (BPTB) autograft has become the most common graft choice for ACL reconstruction and is considered the reference standard [13–15], it also is associated with significant morbidity including quadriceps weakness, patellofemoral pain, loss of motion, patella fracture, patellar tendonitis, patella infera syndrome, early degenerative joint changes, and arthrofibrosis [16–20]. Semitendinosus gracilis autografts have become more popular for ACL reconstruction, with outcomes similar to those of BPTB grafts without the extensor mechanism dysfunction; however, deficits in knee flexor strength, variability in hamstring size, fixation limitations, delayed incorporation, and surgeon experience have affected their overall use [21–30]. As surgeons and patients look for ways to limit the significant morbidity associated with autograft harvest, allograft tissue has become increasingly popular for ACL reconstruction. The senior author (C.D.H.) has noted a significant increase in the use of allograft tissue among his colleagues for ACL reconstruction. Currently allograft tissue is used in approximately 30% of primary ACL reconstructions and in 90% of revision ACL reconstructions in his practice.

Allograft tissue has the advantage of no donor-site morbidity, larger and predictable graft sizes, low incidence of arthrofibrosis, shorter operative time, and

*Corresponding author. Department of Orthopaedic Surgery, Division of Sports Medicine, University of Pittsburgh Medical Center, UPMC Center for Sports Medicine, 3200 S. Water Street, Pittsburgh PA 15203. E-mail address: harnercd@upmc.edu (C.D. Harner).

0278-5919/07/$ – see front matter
doi:10.1016/j.csm.2007.06.010

improved overall health-related quality of life [31]; however, disadvantages including cost, slower incorporation, and potential for bacterial, viral, and prion disease transmission have limited its acceptance for routine ACL reconstruction [13]. Thus, the optimal graft material remains controversial. The optimal graft should be able to reproduce the anatomy and biomechanics of the ACL, be incorporated rapidly with strong initial fixation, and cause low graft-site morbidity. This article reviews the literature comparing the clinical outcomes following allograft and autograft ACL reconstruction and examines current issues regarding graft choice.

CLINICAL OUTCOMES OF AUTOGRAFT VERSUS ALLOGRAFT RECONSTRUCTION

No level I randomized, blinded studies comparing the outcomes of allograft versus autograft ACL reconstruction currently exist in the literature. Graft choice is influenced by the preoperative examination, patient age, activity level, and comorbidities as well as by surgeon preference, experience, and bias. Discussion of graft choice with patients must take into account all of these variables, the risks and benefits of each option, and the patient's preference regarding graft choice. With the inherent risks and benefits of each option, randomization of patients would be very difficult to achieve, because the patient must be part of the decision to use or not use allograft tissue; therefore, a well-designed cohort study probably is the best study that can be performed. During the past 10 years the authors were able to identify 10 cohort studies in the English literature that compare the outcomes following autograft versus allograft ACL reconstruction. Each of these articles is reviewed briefly here (Table 1).

Rihn and colleagues [32] compared the outcomes of 102 patients who underwent ACL reconstruction with either BPTB autograft (63 patients) or BPTB allograft (39 patients) sterilized with 2.5 Mrad of irradiation at an average of 4.2 years of follow-up. They found that patients undergoing allograft reconstruction were significantly older (44 years versus 25 years) and had a longer delay from injury to surgery (17.1 weeks versus 9.7 weeks) but had no difference in International Knee Documentation Committee (IKDC) subjective knee scores (86.7 for allograft versus 88.0 for autograft). Physical examination findings revealed no significant difference in patellofemoral symptoms, range of motion, vertical jump, or single-legged hop tests. Allograft-reconstructed patients had slightly improved side-to-side pivot-shift results (92% equal with allograft versus 74.2% equal with autograft, $P = .06$) and a reduced KT-1000 (MEDmetric Corporation, San Diego, California) maximum manual side-to-side difference (1.3 mm for allograft versus 2.2 mm for autograft; $P = .04$). Overall, approximately 95% of patients receiving allograft reconstructions and 98% of patients receiving autograft reconstructions rated their knee function as normal or nearly normal, and 95% of patients receiving allograft reconstructions and 94% of patients receiving autograft reconstructions rated their activity levels as normal or nearly normal. The authors concluded that similar patient-reported and objective outcomes can be obtained with both autograft and allograft BPTB reconstructions and that a bactericidal dose of 2.5 Mrad of irradiation as a means of graft sterilization did not compromise the clinical outcome.

Poehling and colleagues [33] prospectively compared subjective and objective outcomes of patients undergoing ACL reconstruction with either BPTB autograft (118 patients) or Achilles tendon allograft (41 patients) for up to 5 years of follow-up (average of 4.2 years for subjective measures and 2.2 years for objective measures). Using the Rand 36-item health survey and the McGill Pain Questionnaire, the authors found that patients undergoing allograft reconstruction had significantly improved physical functioning for the first year following surgery, less severe pain for the first 3 months following surgery, and fewer limitations in function throughout the follow-up period. Overall IKDC values showed no differences between autograft and allograft ACL reconstruction except at the 2-year point, when 50% of autograft knees and 89% of allograft knees were rated as normal or nearly normal ($P = .037$). KT-1000 measurement values were less in autograft recipients (2.8 mm versus 3.0 mm allograft; $P = .052$), but side-to-side KT-1000 measurements revealed no difference between autograft and allograft, and the values were found to decrease over the 5-year follow-up period. Additionally, in a related article, the authors reported that analysis of surgical costs data found the mean hospital charge for an ACL reconstruction was $4622 with allograft and $5694 with autograft [34]. The increased cost for autograft reconstruction resulted from increased operating room time and an increased likelihood of overnight hospitalization for pain control with autograft recipients. Despite differences in graft type, fixation, and treating surgeon, the authors concluded that similar long-term results in stability and function were achieved with BPTB autograft and Achilles tendon allograft reconstruction of the ACL, but that patients treated with allograft reconstruction had less pain and functional limitations in the early postoperative period.

Many practices have considered older patient age to be a relative indication for using allograft tissue in ACL reconstruction. Barrett and colleagues [35] examined the clinical outcomes of patients 40 years or older having at least 2 years of follow-up after ACL reconstruction with BPTB autograft or allograft. At final follow-up, subjective evaluation using a 15-question visual analogue scale revealed no difference between patients treated with allograft or autograft. IKDC functional levels were normal or nearly normal in 87% of patients in the allograft group and in 96% of patients in the autograft group. KT-1000 side-to-side differences were 1.46 mm for the allograft group and 0.104 mm for the autograft group. Final follow-up Tegner activity rating scale scores and Lysholm scores did not differ between groups, but allograft-treated patients had a quicker return to activities. There was one clinical failure in the allograft group and none in the autograft group. The authors concluded that allograft reconstruction allows a quicker return to sporting activities but has greater laxity than autograft BPTB reconstruction. They believed that both graft choices were highly effective and that the benefits and disadvantages of each graft

Table 1
Clinical outcome studies of autograft versus allograft anterior cruciate ligament reconstruction

Study	Graft type		Study Type	# Patients		Average age (years)		Follow-up (months)	N/NN IKDC (%)		Laxity (KT 1000)		Functional Differences/ Conclusions
	Auto	Allo		Auto	Allo	Auto	Allo		Auto	Allo	Auto	Allo	
Rihn et al, 2006 [32]	BPTB	BPTB	RR	63	39	25.3	44	50.4	82.70	90.70	2.2 mm	1.3 mm	No functional differences Low-dose irradiation does not affect outcome
Poehling et al, 2005 [33]	BPTB	Achilles	PC	118	41	25.4	29.7	50.4/26.4 (sub/obj)	50 2-year follow-up	89	2.8 mm	3.0 mm	Improved physical function first 2 years allograft less pain for first 6 to 12 months with allograft Functional outcome at 5 years equivalent

Study	Autograft	Allograft	Design	n (auto)	n (allo)	Age (auto)	Age (allo)	Follow-up	Outcome (auto)	Outcome (allo)	Laxity (auto)	Laxity (allo)	Comments
Barrett et al, 2005 [35]	BPTB	BPTB	PC	25	38	44.5	47.1	48.4/36.4 (auto/allo)	96 Functional	87	0.104 mm	1.46 mm	Earlier return to sporting activities with allograft; Increased laxity with allograft; No functional difference
Kustos et al 2004 [36]	BPTB	BPTB	RR	26	53	24.5	25.6	38	No difference in IKDC scores; Average Lysholm scores 89.9	84.1	Slightly > autograft		Loss of full extension more common in autograft; Equivalent functional outcomes
Chang et al, 2003 [37]	BPTB	BPTB Augmented with IT band tenodesis	RR	33	46	28.7	33.1	40/33 (auto/allo)	97 G/E Lysholm scores	90.70	1.1 mm	1.2 mm	Increased flexion deficit with allograft; Slightly improved results with autograft; Allograft reasonable alternative

(continued on next page)

Table 1
(continued)

Study	Graft type		Study Type	# Patients		Average age (years)		Follow-up (months)	N/NN IKDC (%)		Laxity (KT 1000)		Functional Differences/ Conclusions
	Auto	Allo		Auto	Allo	Auto	Allo		Auto	Allo	Auto	Allo	
Peterson et al, 2001 [14] (5-year follow-up of Shelton)	BPTB	BPTB	PC	30	30	25	28	64.6/62.5 (auto/allo)	88.6 Average Lysholm scores	90	67% <3 mm side-to-side	73%	Autograft group had slight extension loss Increased # allograft with glide on pivot shift No functional/ objective difference at 5 years

Study	Graft	Design								Stability	Outcome
Shelton et al, 1997 [38]	BPTB	PC	30	30	25	27	24	Not reported		70% / 73% <3 mm side-to-side	Increased # allograft with glide on pivot shift / No difference between groups at 2 years
Kleipoo et al, 1998 [39]	BPTB	PC	26	36	28	28	52/46 (auto/allo)	70	85	69% / 75% <3 mm side-to-side	No functional differences / Poor results linked to tibial tunnel position
Stringham et al, 1996 [15]	BPTB	RR	47	31	25	26	34	NR		80% / 70% <3 mm side-to-side	Four traumatic ruptures with allograft / Improved AP stability with autograft
Harner et al, 1996 [13]	BPTB	RR	26	64	23.9	45		39	48	1.9 mm / 1.8 mm	No functional differences

Abbreviations: Allo, allograft; auto, autograft; BPTB, bone-patellar tendon-bone; IKDC, International Knee Documentation Committee; N/NN, normal or nearly normal; PC, prospective cohort; RR, retrospective review; sub/oj, subjective/objective; AP, anteroposterior; G/E, good/excellent; IT, iliotibial band.

option should be explained fully to the patients before surgical decision making.

Kustos and colleagues [36] reviewed the results of 79 patients who had undergone ACL reconstruction with either allograft (53 patients) or autograft (26 patients) in a young (25 years) Hungarian population. The patients were followed for an average of 38 months following ACL reconstruction with BPTB grafts secured with interference screws. Both groups had equivalent Lysholm knee scores, Tegner activity scores, and functional IKDC results. Two allograft recipients and one autograft patient suffered a traumatic rupture of the graft. The authors concluded that BPTB allograft is a good alternative to autograft and should be offered to patients as an alternative graft choice.

Chang and colleagues [37] retrospectively reviewed the minimum 2-year outcomes following BPTB allograft versus autograft ACL reconstruction augmented with iliotibial band tenodesis. The allograft group averaged 4.4 years older, had greater preoperative laxity, and had a higher rate of medial tibial plateau chondromalacia than the autograft group. Three allograft recipients suffered traumatic ruptures of the graft more than 1 year postoperatively. Ninety-one percent of the allograft recipients versus 97% of the autograft recipients had good-to-excellent results based on Lysholm II scores. Although the study lacked adequate power for statistical significance, it showed a trend toward better results with autograft reconstruction. Sixty-five percent of the allograft recipients and 73% of the autograft recipients were able to return to preinjury activity levels. Thirty-two percent of allograft recipients and 18% of autograft recipients had a grade I Lachman examination with a firm end point, and 5% of the allograft recipients had a grade I pivot-shift examination. When range of motion was tested, 5% of allograft recipients versus 0% autograft recipients had an extension deficit of at least 5°; 53% of allograft recipients versus 22.7% of autograft recipients had a flexion deficit of at least 5° ($P = .02$). KT-1000 side-to-side measurements did not reveal a difference between groups. The authors concluded that allograft reconstruction is a reasonable alternative to autograft BPTB reconstruction, but the results are not quite as good.

Shelton and colleagues [14,38] prospectively followed a group of 30 allograft and 30 autograft ACL reconstructions for 2 and 5 years. Half of the allograft recipients had chronic injuries (> 6 months at the time of surgery), versus only 20% of the autograft recipients. At 2 years there was no difference in pain, giving way, motion, or patellofemoral crepitus. Eight allograft knees had an increased Lachman examination, compared with five autograft knees, and six allograft knees had a grade 1 pivot-shift compared with two autograft knees. Twenty-nine of 30 allograft recipients and 28 of 30 autograft recipients had a KT-1000 measurement of less than 5 mm. At the 5-year follow-up, the two groups had equivalent Lysholm scores (88.6 autograft versus 90.0 allograft) and Tegner activity scores (6.1 autograft versus 5.4 allograft). There was one traumatic graft rupture in each group. Autograft reconstructed knees had lost 2.5° of extension versus 1.1° in the allograft knees ($P = .027$). Six allograft knees and seven autograft knees had an increased Lachman examination, and four allograft and two autograft knees had an increased pivot-shift examination. Fifty-three percent of autograft recipients and 7% of allograft recipients had incisional-site complaints. The authors concluded that BPTB autograft and allograft ACL reconstruction produced statistically similar results at both 2 and 5 years and that allograft was an acceptable choice for primary ACL reconstruction.

Kleipool and colleagues [39] prospectively followed the results for a group of 62 patients who underwent ACL reconstruction with either fresh-frozen BPTB allograft (36 patients) or autograft (26 patients). The patient populations were similar in age, activity level, and associated injuries. Preoperatively the allograft group had significantly worse Lachman and anterior drawer tests than the the autograft group. At a mean follow-up of 52 months for the autograft group and 46 months for the allograft group, an IKDC rating of normal or nearly normal had been achieved in 70% of the autograft group and 85% of the allograft group. Lysholm scores averaged 95 in the autograft group and 94 in the allograft group. No differences in Lachman, anterior drawer, pivot-shift, one-leg hop test, or KT-1000 side-to-side difference was detected between groups. Mild-to-moderate anterior knee pain was found in 42% of autograft recipients and 53% of allograft recipients. Two autograft recipients had disabling anterior knee pain; no allograft recipients had disabling pain. The investigators did find that anteriorly placed tibial tunnels were associated with poorer outcomes and increased laxity in both autograft and allograft groups. In a related study, Zijl and colleagues [40] found no difference in tunnel enlargement following ACL BPTB reconstruction with either autograft or allograft. Tunnel enlargement did not correlate with clinical outcome, and enlargement of the tunnels was found to decrease with time. These investigators again confirmed that malpositioned tunnels led to poorer clinical outcomes, and they did see a trend of increased tunnel enlargement in anteriorly malpositioned tunnels. The authors concluded from both studies that BPTB allograft was a good alternative to autograft tissue with similar subjective and objective results at 4 years of follow-up and that tunnel positioning is of great importance in preventing poor clinical outcomes.

Stringham and colleagues [15] retrospectively reviewed the results for 78 patients 34 months following ACL reconstruction with BPTB autograft (47 patients) or allograft (31 patients). The two groups of patients were similar in age (25 years), activity level, time from injury to surgery, associated injuries, and type of fixation used on both tibial and femoral sides. Both groups had an equal satisfaction ratings postoperatively, and there was no difference between the two groups in subjective symptoms (pain, instability, swelling, and locking). Objective results showed no difference for joint effusions, knee tenderness, range of motion, quadriceps atrophy, patellofemoral scores, or extension deficits. The authors found two trends in the study that did not reach statistical significance. Eighty percent of autograft recipients versus 70% of allograft recipients achieved good-to-excellent restoration of anteroposterior stability (< 3 mm side-to-side laxity difference), and patients who had undergone allograft reconstruction had increased concentric peak extension torque results at 60°/second. Reconstructions in six patients (four autograft, two allograft) were considered failures because of side-to-side laxity measurements greater than 5 mm. Four traumatic ruptures occurred in patients who had undergone allograft reconstruction at an average of 11 months postoperatively (range, 4–17 months). No traumatic ruptures occurred in the autograft group ($P =$ .011). The authors concluded that, with the increased rate of traumatic ruptures in the allograft group, autograft BPTB was their first choice for ACL reconstruction. When the use of autologous tissue was contraindicated or a knee had multiple ligament injuries, allograft tissue was the preferred graft choice.

In the final study, Harner and colleagues [13] retrospectively reviewed the clinical outcomes of 64 patients who had undergone allograft BPTB ACL reconstruction and 26 patients who had undergone autograft BPTB ACL reconstruction at 3 to 5 years postoperatively. At latest follow-up, 65% of autograft recipients and 58% of allograft recipients returned to the same or higher level of sports participation, with 54% of patients who had had autograft reconstructions and 56% of patients who had had allograft reconstructions returning to the same or a more stressful sport. Of the patients not returning to the same level of sport, 45% of autograft recipients and 68% of allograft recipients attributed the decreased level of sports participation to factors other than the knee (work, family, school, or other considerations). Fifty-eight percent and 48% of allograft recipients reported no limitations with jumping/landing or cutting/pivoting, respectively, whereas only 39% and 35% of autograft recipients had no problems with jumping/landing and cutting/pivoting, respectively. Sixty-nine percent of autograft recipients and 84% of allograft recipients had no pain with moderate or strenuous activities. Autograft recipients had a mean loss of 3° of active extension and 3.6° loss of passive extension, compared with 1.2° active and 1.3° passive extension loss for allograft recipients ($P <$. 05) although clinically the limited loss probably is not significant. No significant differences were found for KT-1000 laxity testing, pivot-shift, reverse pivot-shift, posterior drawer, varus opening, and valgus opening. The average vertical jump index was 95% for autograft recipients and 91% for allograft recipients; the average one-legged hop index was 98% for autograft recipients and 92% for allograft recipients. The overall IKDC rating was normal or nearly normal for 38% of autograft recipients compared with 48% of allograft recipients. The authors concluded that there were no significant clinical differences in outcome between patients who had undergone autograft BPTB reconstruction versus allograft BPTB ACL reconstruction.

DISEASE TRANSMISSION AND INFECTION

The risk of disease transmission and infection is an important factor when weighing the options of allograft versus autograft ACL reconstruction. Three cases of viral disease transmission have been reported following ACL reconstruction with BPTB allograft: a single case of HIV transmission was reported in 1985, and two cases of hepatitis C were reported in 1991 [41–43]. This risk of disease transmission, especially for HIV, is one of the first questions that most patients and family members raise when the topic of using allograft tissue is raised. Because of this concern, donor selection and screening has been emphasized as a crucial first step in assuring the safety of allograft tissue. The American Association of Tissue Banks recommends serologic screening for human HIV, human T-cell leukemia virus, hepatitis B, hepatitis C, aerobic and anaerobic bacteria, and syphilis as well as harvesting allograft tissue within 12 hours of cold ischemia time [44,45]. Many tissue banks perform polymerase chain reaction testing for HIV to help lower the risk of HIV transmission. When these steps are combined with freezing of the allograft tissue, the estimated risk for HIV transmission with connective tissue allografts is estimated to be 1:8,000,000 [46]. Individual tissue banks differ in their methods of procurement, testing, and processing, and therefore the surgeon should be familiar and comfortable with the methods used.

Bacterial infection following allograft ACL reconstruction is another major concern for patients, families, and physicians. In 2002, the Centers for Disease Control and Prevention (CDC) reported 26 cases allograft-associated bacterial infections in an estimated 1 million allografts distributed for transplantation [47]. Thirteen of the infections, including one death, were associated with *Clostridium* spp. The source of the infection in eight of these cases was contaminated frozen tendons used for ACL reconstruction. Of the remaining 13 cases, 11 were infected with gram-negative bacilli, 5 of which were polymicrobial, and 2 patients had negative cultures. Ten of these 13 cases involved frozen tissue used for ACL reconstruction. The CDC identified 14 of the cases as associated with a single tissue processor. The CDC made specific recommendations to tissue banks to decrease the risk of bacterial contamination: culturing tissue before suspension in antimicrobial solutions, validating culture methods to eliminate false-negative culture results, performing both destructive and swab cultures, and limiting the time between death, refrigeration, and tissue retrieval. The CDC went on to recommend using sterilization techniques including gamma irradiation or sporicidal techniques when applicable to the graft source. Barbour and colleagues [48] reported on four additional cases of *Clostridium septicum* infection following ACL reconstruction between 1998 and 2001. Again, the transmission of disease was linked to tissue procurement and processing. Two large studies examined postoperative infection following ACL reconstruction with either autograft or allograft tissue. In the first report, Williams and colleagues [49] reviewed 2500 ACL reconstructions, 7 (0.3%) of which became infected. In a more recent report, Indelli and colleagues [50] reviewed the infection rate following 3500 ACL reconstructions (60% allograft) performed at Stanford University between 1992 and 1998. They found a deep infection rate of 0.14%, with only two of six infections occurring in allograft-reconstructed knees. No difference in infection rates existed between allograft and autograft ACL reconstructions. These studies, as well as the reports from the CDC, indicate that there is no increased risk for bacterial infection with allograft tissue as long as the tissue bank undertakes preventive measures in procuring and processing of graft tissue.

Allograft tissue can be used for fresh grafts or preserved by three main methods: cryopreserved, fresh-frozen, or freeze-dried. Fresh grafts are maintained in lactated Ringer's solution at 4°C for up to 7 days. Fresh grafts maintain cell viability, but the short time frame available for accurate serologic testing limits their use in clinical practice. Cryopreservation uses a controlled rate of freezing with a cryoprotectant media to maintain cell viability. Studies have found that 10% to 40% of cells in cryopreserved soft tissue grafts maintain viability [51]. The importance of donor-cell viability is questioned in ACL reconstruction, however. Several studies have demonstrated the rapid repopulation of allograft tissue with host cells within 4 weeks of transplantation [52,53], and results using cryopreserved tissues have not been superior to those for fresh-frozen allograft tissue [42]. Fresh-frozen tissues are stored at −80°C, are simple and less expensive to prepare than cryopreserved or freeze-dried grafts, and lack donor-cell viability. The success of ACL reconstruction with fresh-frozen grafts, as well as their ease of preparation and storage, has made fresh-frozen tissue the most common grafts used for soft tissue reconstruction [42,48]. Freeze-dried allograft tissue also is commonly used. Freeze-drying involves dehydration of graft tissue during freezing in a vacuum. Freeze-drying alters the color, appearance, and strength of the graft but allows extended storage at room temperature [42,48]. Results of ACL reconstruction with freeze-dried grafts have been mixed. Indelicato and colleagues [54] found that patients receiving fresh-frozen grafts faired slightly better than patients receiving freeze-dried grafts. Several other studies have found successful clinical outcomes following ACL reconstruction with freeze-dried tissue (see the article by Mahirogullari and colleagues in this issue) [55,56].

Secondary sterilization methods such as ethylene oxide or gamma irradiation may be used to decrease the risk of bacterial or viral transmission. Ethylene oxide treatment has been used with a wide variety of biologic tissues, but several studies have shown problems in tendon allografts with graft dissolution, synovial effusions, and poor clinical outcomes [57,58]. Therefore its use is not recommended for ligament reconstruction. Gamma irradiation also has been used for secondary sterilization. Gamma irradiation neutralizes both viruses and bacteria by direct destruction of the organism's genome and through free-radical production. Many tissue banks irradiate tissues with 1.5- to 2.5-Mrad doses. These doses are effective at destroying many micro-organisms, but recent studies have shown that doses as high as 4 Mrad are required to neutralize HIV from BPTB allografts [59]. Schwartz and colleagues [60] demonstrated in a goat model that a 4-Mrad dose of gamma irradiation had a significant negative effect on allograft tissue load relaxation, stiffness, and maximum force compared with controls at zero and 6 months postoperatively. Other studies have shown that doses of gamma irradiation as low as 2 Mrad have deleterious effects on the initial strength and stiffness of soft tissue allografts [59,61–66]. Several studies, however, have demonstrated that doses less than 2.5 Mrad have no effect on ACL reconstruction [32,67]. Because of the detrimental effects of high-dose gamma irradiation on allograft tissue, it currently is recommended that detailed donor screening, aseptic harvesting and cleaning, antibiotic washes, and multiple aerobic and anaerobic bacterial cultures, with or without low-dose irradiation (< 2.5 Mrad), is the best technique to produce allograft tissue with low risk for disease transmission [42].

GRAFT BIOMECHANICAL PROPERTIES AND INCORPORATION

Autograft ACL reconstruction most commonly is performed using a BPTB graft. The use of quadrupled hamstring tendon has increased in recent years, and a small percentage of surgeons use quadriceps tendon [68]. Various studies have evaluated the biomechanical properties of graft material used for ACL reconstruction (Table 2). The native ACL has been found to have an ultimate tensile load of approximately 2160 newtons (N), a stiffness of 242 N/mm, and a cross-sectional area of 44 mm^2 [69–71]. BPTB grafts (10 mm) were found to have an ultimate tensile load of 2977 N, a stiffness of 620 N/mm, and a cross-sectional area of 35 mm^2 [72]. Biomechanical properties for quadrupled hamstring and quadriceps tendon (10 mm) have found ultimate tensile loads of 4090 N and 2174 N, stiffness of 776 N/mm and 463 N/mm, and cross-sectional areas of 53 mm^2 and 62 mm^2, respectively [73–75]. Other grafts that are used commonly for allograft ACL reconstruction include tibialis anterior, tibialis posterior, and Achilles tendon. Biomechanical studies have found ultimate tensile loads of up to 4122 N and 3594 N, stiffness up to 460 N/mm and 379 N/mm, and cross-sectional areas of 48.2 mm^2 and 44.4 mm^2 for doubled tibialis anterior and tibialis posterior grafts, respectively [76,77]. Achilles tendon grafts have shown ultimate failure loads of 4617 N, stiffness of 685 N/mm, and cross-sectional area of 67 mm^2 [78,79]. The findings from these studies indicate that the grafts commonly used for autograft and allograft ACL reconstruction have similar biomechanical properties and compare favorably with the intact ACL. Woo and colleagues [80] and Smith and colleagues [81] demonstrated that freezing and storage have minimal effect on the ultimate tensile strength and load-deformation mechanics of tendons and ligaments. Furthermore, Pearsall and colleagues [77] demonstrated that tendons from older donors had biomechanical properties similar to those of tendons harvested from younger individuals, increasing the potential donor pool for soft tissue grafts. Clinical outcome studies have supported the use of allograft tissue for ACL reconstructions with rates of excellent and good results comparable to those achieved with autograft reconstruction [13–15,32,33,35–40,54–56,82–90].

The incorporation of graft tissue is another important consideration when evaluating graft choice and timing for return to sport. All grafts, whether autograft or allograft, undergo a sequential process of healing and "ligamentization" consisting of inflammation and graft necrosis, revascularization and cell repopulation, and remodeling [91–97]. The first phase begins nearly immediately after implantation, may continue for the first 1 to 2 months after surgery, and involves an inflammatory response in which the donor fibroblasts undergo cell death and the remaining collagenous tissue becomes a scaffold for subsequent remodeling [91,97]. The second phase of graft incorporation involves

Table 2
Comparison of autograft and allograft tissue options for anterior cruciate ligament reconstruction

Graft type	Ultimate tensile load (N)	Stiffness (N/mm)	Cross-sectional area (mm²)	Incorporation	Method of fixation	Morbidity
Native ACL [69–71]	2160	242	44	NA	NA	NA
BPTB auto (10 mm) [72]	2977	455	32	Bone-to-bone 6 weeks	Interference screws	Anterior knee pain Large incision Quadriceps weakness
Hamstring auto (quadrupled) [73]	4090	776	53	Soft tissue 12 weeks	Variable options	Hamstring weakness
Quadriceps tendon auto [74,75] (10 mm)	2174	463	62	Bone-to-bone and soft tissue (6–12 weeks)	Variable options	Anterior knee pain Quadriceps weakness
BPTB allo (10 mm) [72]	2977	620	35	Bone-to-bone delayed compared with Auto > 6 months	Interference screws	NA
Hamstring allo (quadrupled) [73]	4090	776	53	Soft tissue delayed compared with Auto > 6 months	Variable options	NA
Tibialis anterior (doubled) [76,77]	4122	460	48.2	Soft tissue delayed > 6 months	Variable options	NA
Tibialis posterior (doubled) [76,77]	3594	379	44.4	Soft tissue delayed > 6 months	Variable options	NA
Achilles tendon [78,79]	4617	685	67	Bone-to-bone and soft tissue delayed > 6 months	Variable options	NA

Abbreviations: ACL, anterior cruciate ligament; allo, allograft; auto, autograft; N, newtons; NA, not applicable.

revascularization and migration of host fibroblasts into the graft tissue, typically begins within 20 days of surgery, and may continue throughout the first 6 months following surgery [52,91,94,97,98]. During this phase of graft maturation, changes occur in the material properties of the graft. Graft strength may drop to as low as 11% of the normal ACL during this phase [95], emphasizing the need for protected rehabilitation during this period. During the final phase of graft healing, the graft undergoes maturation and remodeling. The microvascularity, cellular population, and collagen bundle orientation in the replacement tissue matures fully to a nearly normal ACL appearance within 12 to 18 months postoperatively [94,99–102]. The biomechanical properties of the graft material also improve during the final phase of remodeling but do not recover to the initial stiffness and strength of the material at the time of implantation [91,93,95,103].

Healing of the graft material to the tunnel wall is another important consideration when evaluating graft choices. Bone-to-bone healing, as occurs with BPTB grafts, is relatively quick, with incorporation into the host bone often seen by 6 weeks. Soft tissue-to-bone incorporation takes considerably longer, often taking 8 to 12 weeks to mature [96]. Additionally, incorporation of allograft tissue occurs at a slower rate than autograft tissue. Jackson and colleagues [93] found, in a goat model, that allograft BPTB grafts demonstrated a prolonged inflammatory stage, smaller cross-sectional area, delayed remodeling of collagen fibers, and decreased mechanical strength for the first 6 months after reconstruction. Zhang and colleagues [104] demonstrated, in a dog soft tissue reconstruction model, that at 6 months the maturation of the insertional bone–tendon interface was delayed in allograft tissue in comparison with autograft tissue. Nikolaou and colleagues [105], however, found, in a dog model, that by 24 weeks autograft and allograft tissue had nearly normal revascularization and by 36 weeks the mechanical properties of autograft and allograft tissue were similar and had approached 90% of the control ligament strength. Shino and colleagues [100] and Yamagishi and colleagues [106] found that mature revascularization takes 18 months to occur for both autograft and allograft ACL reconstruction. These differences in graft incorporation and maturation between bone and soft tissue grafts and between autograft and allograft may be important factors to consider when determining rehabilitation criteria and timing for return to play.

SUMMARY

ACL reconstruction is one of the procedures most commonly performed by sports medicine physicians today. Good-to-excellent results in terms of knee stability, patient satisfaction, and return to athletic activity are reported commonly to be around 90% [107]. Although BPTB grafts traditionally have been considered the reference standard, donor-site morbidity has led to an interest in alternative graft choices. Commonly used autograft options to BPTB include hamstring tendons and, to a far lesser extent, quadriceps tendon grafts. Allograft options include BPTB, Achilles tendon, anterior and posterior tibialis grafts, hamstring tendons, and fascia lata grafts. With successful clinical outcomes achieved with both autograft and allograft tissues, the choice of graft material becomes one of surgeon and patient preference. Autograft tissue offers the advantages of no risk of disease transmission, a high success rate, and no immunogenic response. These benefits must be balanced with donor-site morbidity, difficulty of graft harvest, additional operating room time associated with graft harvest, and the limits and unpredictability in graft size and quality. Allograft tissue has the advantages of lacking donor-site morbidity, smaller incisions, decreased operative time, easier and less painful rehabilitation, and larger and more predictable graft sizes. The major disadvantage of allograft reconstruction is the risk of disease transmission; although with current screening, processing, and sterilization techniques the risk is extremely low, it should not be overlooked. Additionally, when using allograft tissue, one must be aware that allograft tissue may generate a low-level immune response. It also has been shown to have delayed incorporation time, and the cost for the allograft tissue itself is greater. Overall, no graft choice can match completely the characteristics and function of the native ACL. The ideal graft choice should have biomechanical properties similar to those of the native ACL, have low morbidity, incorporate quickly, and be able to restore functional stability to the knee over the long term while taking into account individual patient factors, including patient preference, activity level, prior surgery, comorbidities, and goals.

References

[1] Muneta T, Sekiya I, Yagishita K, et al. Two-bundle reconstruction of the anterior cruciate ligament using semitendinosus tendon with EndoButtons: operative technique and preliminary results. Arthroscopy 1999;15(6):618–24.
[2] Ireland ML. Anterior cruciate ligament injury in female athletes: epidemiology. J Athl Train 1999;34(2):150–4.
[3] Arendt E, Dick R. Knee injury patterns among men and women in collegiate basketball and soccer. NCAA data and review of literature. Am J Sports Med 1995;23(6):694–701.
[4] Arendt EA, Agel J, Dick R. Anterior cruciate ligament injury patterns among collegiate men and women. J Athl Train 1999;34(2):86–92.
[5] Fu FH, Bennett CH, Lattermann C, et al. Current trends in anterior cruciate ligament reconstruction. Part 1: biology and biomechanics of reconstruction. Am J Sports Med 1999;27(6):821–30.
[6] Ireland ML. The female ACL: why is it more prone to injury? Orthop Clin North Am 2002;33(4):637–51.
[7] Shelbourne KD, Patel DV. Timing of surgery in anterior cruciate ligament-injured knees. Knee Surg Sports Traumatol Arthrosc 1995;3(3):148–56.
[8] Soderman K, Pietila T, Alfredson H, et al. Anterior cruciate ligament injuries in young females playing soccer at senior levels. Scand J Med Sci Sports 2002;12(2):65–8.
[9] American Board of Orthopaedic Surgery. Research committee report: diplomatic newsletter. Chapel Hill (NC): American Board of Orthopaedic Surgery; 2004.
[10] Brown CH Jr, Carson EW. Revision anterior cruciate ligament surgery. Clin Sports Med 1999;18(1):109–71.
[11] Harner CD, Giffin JR, Dunteman RC, et al. Evaluation and treatment of recurrent instability after anterior cruciate ligament reconstruction. Instr Course Lect 2001;50:463–74.
[12] Harner CD, Poehling GG. Double bundle or double trouble? Arthroscopy 2004;20(10):1013–4.

[13] Harner CD, Olson E, Irrgang JJ, et al. Allograft versus autograft anterior cruciate ligament reconstruction: 3- to 5-year outcome. Clin Orthop Relat Res 1996;324:134–44.

[14] Peterson RK, Shelton WR, Bomboy AL. Allograft versus autograft patellar tendon anterior cruciate ligament reconstruction: a 5-year follow-up. Arthroscopy 2001;17(1): 9–13.

[15] Stringham DR, Pelmas CJ, Burks RT, et al. Comparison of anterior cruciate ligament reconstructions using patellar tendon autograft or allograft. Arthroscopy 1996;12(4): 414–21.

[16] Aglietti P, Buzzi R, D'Andria S, et al. Patellofemoral problems after intraarticular anterior cruciate ligament reconstruction. Clin Orthop Relat Res 1993;288:195–204.

[17] Kleipool AE, van Loon T, Marti RK. Pain after use of the central third of the patellar tendon for cruciate ligament reconstruction. 33 patients followed 2–3 years. Acta Orthop Scand 1994;65(1):62–6.

[18] Sachs RA, Daniel DM, Stone ML, et al. Patellofemoral problems after anterior cruciate ligament reconstruction. Am J Sports Med 1989;17(6):760–5.

[19] Marumoto JM, Mitsunaga MM, Richardson AB, et al. Late patellar tendon ruptures after removal of the central third for anterior cruciate ligament reconstruction. A report of two cases. Am J Sports Med 1996;24(5):698–701.

[20] Snyder-Mackler L, Delitto A, Bailey SL, et al. Strength of the quadriceps femoris muscle and functional recovery after reconstruction of the anterior cruciate ligament. A prospective, randomized clinical trial of electrical stimulation. J Bone Joint Surg Am 1995;77(8): 1166–73.

[21] Maeda A, Shino K, Horibe S, et al. Anterior cruciate ligament reconstruction with multi-stranded autogenous semitendinosus tendon. Am J Sports Med 1996;24(4):504–9.

[22] Yasuda K, Tsujino J, Ohkoshi Y, et al. Graft site morbidity with autogenous semitendinosus and gracilis tendons. Am J Sports Med 1995;23(6):706–14.

[23] Hiemstra LA, Webber S, MacDonald PB, et al. Knee strength deficits after hamstring tendon and patellar tendon anterior cruciate ligament reconstruction. Med Sci Sports Exerc 2000;32(8):1472–9.

[24] Hiemstra LA, Webber S, MacDonald PB, et al. Hamstring and quadriceps strength balance in normal and hamstring anterior cruciate ligament-reconstructed subjects. Clin J Sport Med 2004;14(5):274–80.

[25] Keays SL, Bullock-Saxton J, Keays AC, et al. Muscle strength and function before and after anterior cruciate ligament reconstruction using semitendonosus and gracilis. Knee 2001;8(3):229–34.

[26] Nakamura N, Horibe S, Sasaki S, et al. Evaluation of active knee flexion and hamstring strength after anterior cruciate ligament reconstruction using hamstring tendons. Arthroscopy 2002;18(6):598–602.

[27] Adachi N, Ochi M, Uchio Y, et al. Harvesting hamstring tendons for ACL reconstruction influences postoperative hamstring muscle performance. Arch Orthop Trauma Surg 2003;123(9):460–5.

[28] Tashiro T, Kurosawa H, Kawakami A, et al. Influence of medial hamstring tendon harvest on knee flexor strength after anterior cruciate ligament reconstruction. A detailed evaluation with comparison of single- and double-tendon harvest. Am J Sports Med 2003;31(4):522–9.

[29] Segawa H, Omori G, Koga Y, et al. Rotational muscle strength of the limb after anterior cruciate ligament reconstruction using semitendinosus and gracilis tendon. Arthroscopy 2002;18(2):177–82.

[30] Viola RW, Sterett WI, Newfield D, et al. Internal and external tibial rotation strength after anterior cruciate ligament reconstruction using ipsilateral semitendinosus and gracilis tendon autografts. Am J Sports Med 2000;28(4):552–5.

[31] Olsen EJ. Use of soft tissue allografts in sports medicine. Advances Operative Orthopaedics 1993;1:111–28.

[32] Rihn JA, Irrgang JJ, Chhabra A, et al. Does irradiation affect the clinical outcome of patellar tendon allograft ACL reconstruction? Knee Surg Sports Traumatol Arthrosc 2006;14(9):885–96.

[33] Poehling GG, Curl WW, Lee CA, et al. Analysis of outcomes of anterior cruciate ligament repair with 5-year follow-up: allograft versus autograft. Arthroscopy 2005;21(7):774–85.

[34] Cole DW, Ginn TA, Chen GJ, et al. Cost comparison of anterior cruciate ligament reconstruction: autograft versus allograft. Arthroscopy 2005;1(7):786–90.

[35] Barrett G, Stokes D, White M. Anterior cruciate ligament reconstruction in patients older than 40 years: allograft versus autograft patellar tendon. Am J Sports Med 2005;33(10):1505–12.

[36] Kustos T, Balint L, Than P, et al. Comparative study of autograft or allograft in primary anterior cruciate ligament reconstruction. Int Orthop 2004;28(5):290–3.

[37] Chang SK, Egami DK, Shaieb MD, et al. Anterior cruciate ligament reconstruction: allograft versus autograft. Arthroscopy 2003;19(5):453–62.

[38] Shelton WR, Papendick L, Dukes AD. Autograft versus allograft anterior cruciate ligament reconstruction. Arthroscopy 1997;13(4):446–9.

[39] Kleipool AE, Zijl JA, Willems WJ. Arthroscopic anterior cruciate ligament reconstruction with bone-patellar tendon-bone allograft or autograft. A prospective study with an average follow up of 4 years. Knee Surg Sports Traumatol Arthrosc 1998;6(4):224–30.

[40] Zijl JA, Kleipool AE, Willems WJ. Comparison of tibial tunnel enlargement after anterior cruciate ligament reconstruction using patellar tendon autograft or allograft. Am J Sports Med 2000;28(4):547–51.

[41] Tomford WW. Transmission of disease through transplantation of musculoskeletal allografts: current concepts review. J Bone Joint Surg Am 1995;77-A:1742–54.

[42] Shelton WR, Treacy SH, Dukes AD, et al. Use of allografts in knee reconstruction: I. Basic science aspects and current status. J Am Acad Orthop Surg 1998;6:165–8.

[43] Simonds RJ, Holmberg SD, Hurwitz RL, et al. Transmission of human immunodeficiency virus type 1 from a seronegative organ and tissue donor. N Engl J Med 1992;326:726–32.

[44] Cole BJ, Carter TR, Rodeo SA. Allograft meniscal transplantation: background, techniques, and results. Instr Course Lect 2003;52:383–96.

[45] Verdonk R, Kohn D. Harvest and conservation of meniscal allografts. Scand J Med Sci Sports 1999;9(3):158–9.

[46] Buck BE, Resnick L, Shah SM, et al. Human immunodeficiency virus cultured from bone. Implications for transplantation. Clin Orthop Relat Res 1990;251:249–53.

[47] Archibald LK, Jernigan DB, Kainer MA. Update: Allograft-associated bacterial infections—United States, 2002. MMWR Morb Mortal Wkly Rep 2002;51(10):207–10.

[48] Barbour SA, King W. The safe and effective use of allograft tissue—an update. Am J Sports Med 2003;31(5):791–7.

[49] Williams RJ, Laurencin CT, Warren RF, et al. Septic arthritis after arthroscopic anterior cruciate ligament reconstruction: diagnosis and management. Am J Sports Med 1997;25(2):261–7.

[50] Indelli PF, Dillingham M, Fanton G, et al. Septic arthritis in postoperative anterior cruciate ligament reconstruction. Clin Orthop Relat Res 2002;398:182–8.

[51] Jackson DW, Whelan J, Simon TM. Cell survival after transplantation of fresh meniscal allografts. DNA probe analysis in a goat model. Am J Sports Med 1993;21(4):540–50.

[52] Jackson DW, Simon TM. Donor cell survival and repopulation after intraarticular transplantation of tendon and ligament allografts. Microsc Res Tech 2002;58(1):25–33.

[53] Goertzen MJ, Buitkamp J, Clahsen H, et al. Cell survival following bone-anterior cruciate ligament-bone allograft transplantation: DNA fingerprints, segregation, and collagen morphological analysis of multiple markers in the canine model. Arch Orthop Trauma Surg 1998;117(4–5):208–14.

[54] Indelicato PA, Bittar ES, Prevot TJ, et al. Clinical comparison of freeze-dried and fresh frozen patellar tendon allografts for anterior cruciate ligament reconstruction of the knee. Am J Sports Med 1990;18(4):335–42.
[55] Levitt RL, Malinin T, Posada A, et al. Reconstruction of anterior cruciate ligaments with bone-patellar tendon-bone and Achilles tendon allografts. Clin Orthop Relat Res 1994;303:67–78.
[56] Noyes FR, Barber-Westin SD. Reconstruction of the anterior cruciate ligament with human allograft. Comparison of early and later results. J Bone Joint Surg Am 1996;78(4):524–37.
[57] Roberts TS, Drez D Jr, McCarthy W, et al. Anterior cruciate ligament reconstruction using freeze-dried, ethylene oxide-sterilized, bone-patellar tendon-bone allografts. Two year results in thirty-six patients. Am J Sports Med 1991;19(1):35–41.
[58] Jackson DW, Windler GE, Simon TM. Intraarticular reaction associated with the use of freeze-dried, ethylene oxide-sterilized bone-patella tendon-bone allografts in the reconstruction of the anterior cruciate ligament. Am J Sports Med 1990;18(1):1–10, [discussion: 10–11].
[59] Fideler BM, Vangsness CT Jr, Lu B, et al. Gamma irradiation: effects on biomechanical properties of human bone-patellar tendon-bone allografts. Am J Sports Med 1995;23(5):643–6.
[60] Schwartz HE, Matava MJ, Proch FS, et al. The effect of gamma irradiation on anterior cruciate ligament allograft biomechanical and biochemical properties in the caprine model at time zero and at 6 months after surgery. Am J Sports Med 2006;34(11):1747–55.
[61] Salehpour A, Butler DL, Proch FS. Dose-dependent response of gamma irradiation on mechanical properties of goat bone-patellar tendon-bone allografts. Transactions Orthopaedic Research Society 1994;19:557.
[62] Curran AR, Adams DJ, Gill JL, et al. The biomechanical effects of low-dose irradiation on bone-patellar tendon-bone allografts. Am J Sports Med 2004;32(5):1131–5.
[63] De Deyne P, Haut RC. Some effects of gamma irradiation on patellar tendon allografts. Connect Tissue Res 1991;27:51–62.
[64] Meeker I, Gross RE. Low-temperature sterilization of organic tissue by high-voltage cathod ray irradiation. Science 1951;114:283–5.
[65] Salehpour A, Butler DL, Proch FS, et al. Dose-dependent response of gamma irradiation on mechanical properties and related biochemical composition of goat bone-patellar tendon-bone allografts. J Orthop Res 1995;13:898–906.
[66] Rasmussen TJ, Feder SM, Butler DL, et al. The effects of 4 Mrad of gamma irradiation on the initial mechanical properties of bone-patellar tendon-bone grafts. Arthroscopy 1994;10(2):188–97.
[67] Butler DL, Oster DM, Feder SM, et al. Effects of gamma irradiation on the biomechanics of patellar tendon allografts of the ACL of the goat. Transactions Orthopaedic Research Society 1991;16:205.
[68] Delay BS, Smolinski RJ, Wind WM, et al. Current practices and opinions in ACL reconstruction and rehabilitation: results of a survey of the American Orthopaedic Society for Sports Medicine. Am J Knee Surg 2001;14(2):85–91.
[69] Woo SL, Hollis JM, Adams DJ, et al. Tensile properties of the human femur-anterior cruciate ligament-tibia complex: the effects of specimen age and orientation. Am J Sports Med 1991;19:217–25.
[70] Noyes FR, Butler DL, Grood ES, et al. Biomechanical analysis of human ligament grafts used in knee-ligament repairs and reconstructions. J Bone Joint Surg Am 1984;66(3):344–52.
[71] Frank CB, Jackson DW. The science of reconstruction of the anterior cruciate ligament. J Bone Joint Surg Am 1997;79:1556–76.
[72] Cooper DE, Deng XH, Burstein AH, et al. The strength of the central third patellar tendon graft: a biomechanical study. Am J Sports Med 1993;21(6):818–23.

[73] Hamner DL Jr, Brown CH, Steiner ME, et al. Hamstring tendon grafts for reconstruction of the anterior cruciate ligament: biomechanical evaluation of the use of multiple strands and tensioning techniques. J Bone Joint Surg Am 1999;81(4):549–57.

[74] Staubli HU, Schatzmann L, Brunner P, et al. Mechanical tensile properties of the quadriceps tendon and patellar ligament in young adults. Am J Sports Med 1999;27(1):27–34.

[75] Harris NL, Smith DA, Lamoreaux L, et al. Central quadriceps tendon for anterior cruciate ligament reconstruction. Part I: morphometric and biomechanical evaluation. Am J Sports Med 1997;25(1):23–8.

[76] Haut Donahue TL, Howell SM, Hull ML, et al. A biomechanical evaluation of anterior and posterior tibialis tendons as suitable single-loop anterior cruciate ligament grafts. Arthroscopy 2002;18(6):589–97.

[77] Pearsall AW, Hollis JM, Russell GV Jr, et al. A biomechanical comparison of three lower extremity tendons for ligamentous reconstruction about the knee. Arthroscopy 2003; 19(10):1091–6.

[78] Wren TAL, Yerby SA, Beaupre GS, et al. Mechanical properties of the human Achilles tendon. Clin Biomech 2001;16:245–51.

[79] Lewis G, Shaw KM. Tensile properties of human tendo Achilles: effect of donor age and strain rate. J Foot Ankle Surg 1997;36(6):435–45.

[80] Woo SL, Orlando CA, Camp JF, et al. Effects of postmortem storage by freezing on ligament tensile behavior. J Biomech 1986;19:399–404.

[81] Smith CW, Young IS, Kearney JN. Mechanical properties of tendons: changes with sterilization and preservation. J Biomech Eng 1996;118:56–61.

[82] Indelicato PA, Linton RC, Huegel M. The results of fresh-frozen patellar tendon allografts for chronic anterior cruciate ligament deficiency of the knee. Am J Sports Med 1992;20(2): 118–21.

[83] Linn RM, Fischer DA, Smith JP, et al. Achilles tendon allograft reconstruction of the anterior cruciate ligament-deficient knee. Am J Sports Med 1993;21(6):825–31.

[84] Nin JR, Leyes M, Schweitzer D. Anterior cruciate ligament reconstruction with fresh-frozen patellar tendon allografts: sixty cases with 2 years' minimum follow-up. Knee Surg Sports Traumatol Arthrosc 1996;4(3):137–42.

[85] Shino K, Nakata K, Horibe S, et al. Quantitative evaluation after arthroscopic anterior cruciate ligament reconstruction. Allograft versus autograft. Am J Sports Med 1993;21(4): 609–16.

[86] Shino K, Inoue M, Horibe S, et al. Reconstruction of the anterior cruciate ligament using allogenic tendon. Long-term followup. Am J Sports Med 1990;18(5):457–65.

[87] Than P, Balint L, Doman I, et al. Replacement of the anterior cruciate ligament of the knee with deep frozen bone-tendon-bone allografts. Ann Transplant 1999;4(3–4):64–7.

[88] Nyland J, Caborn DN, Rothbauer J, et al. Two-year outcomes following ACL reconstruction with allograft tibialis anterior tendons: a retrospective study. Knee Surg Sports Traumatol Arthrosc 2003;11(4):212–8.

[89] Bach BR Jr, Aadalen KJ, Dennis MG, et al. Primary anterior cruciate ligament reconstruction using fresh-frozen, nonirradiated patellar tendon allograft: minimum 2-year follow-up. Am J Sports Med 2005;33(2):284–92.

[90] Fox JA, Pierce M, Bojchuk J, et al. Revision anterior cruciate ligament reconstruction with nonirradiated fresh-frozen patellar tendon allograft. Arthroscopy 2004;20(8):787–94.

[91] Clancy WG Jr, Narechania RG, Rosenberg TD, et al. Anterior and posterior cruciate ligament reconstruction in rhesus monkeys. J Bone Joint Surg Am 1981;63(8):1270–84.

[92] Jackson DW, Corsetti J, Simon TM. Biologic incorporation of allograft anterior cruciate ligament replacements. Clin Orthop Relat Res 1996;324:126–33.

[93] Jackson DW, Grood ES, Goldstein JD, et al. A comparison of patellar tendon autograft and allograft used for anterior cruciate ligament reconstruction in the goat model. Am J Sports Med 1993;21(2):176–85.

[94] Falconiero RP, DiStefano VJ, Cook TM. Revascularization and ligamentization of autogenous anterior cruciate ligament grafts in humans. Arthroscopy 1998;14:197–205.

[95] Beynnon BD, Johnson RJ. Anterior cruciate ligament injury rehabilitation in athletes: biomechanical considerations. Sports Med 1996;22:54–64.

[96] Rodeo SA, Arnoczky SP, Torzilli PA, et al. Tendon-healing in a bone tunnel: a biomechanical and histological study in the dog. J Bone Joint Surg Am 1993;75:1795–803.

[97] Arnoczky SP, Tarvin GB, Marshall JL. Anterior cruciate ligament replacement using patellar tendon. An evaluation of graft revascularization in the dog. J Bone Joint Surg Am 1982;64(2):217–24.

[98] Jackson DW, Grood ES, Arnoczky SP, et al. Freeze dried anterior cruciate ligament allografts. Preliminary studies in a goat model. Am J Sports Med 1987;15(4):295–303.

[99] Jackson DW, Simon TM, Lowery W, et al. Biologic remodeling after anterior cruciate ligament reconstruction using a collagen matrix derived from demineralized bone. An experimental study in the goat model. Am J Sports Med 1996;24(4):405–14.

[100] Shino K, Inoue M, Horibe S, et al. Surface blood flow and histology of human anterior cruciate ligament allografts. Arthroscopy 1991;7(2):171–6.

[101] Shino K. Reconstruction of the anterior cruciate ligament using allogeneic tissues: overview and current practice. Bull Hosp Jt Dis Orthop Inst 1991;51(2):155–74.

[102] Shino K, Inoue M, Nakamura H, et al. Arthroscopic follow-up of anterior cruciate ligament reconstruction using allogeneic tendon. Arthroscopy 1989;5(3):165–71.

[103] Beynnon BD, Johnson RJ, Abate JA, et al. Treatment of anterior cruciate ligament injuries, part 2. Am J Sports Med 2005;33(11):1751–67.

[104] Zhang CL, Fan HB, Xu H, et al. Histological comparison of fate of ligamentous insertion after reconstruction of anterior cruciate ligament: autograft vs allograft. Chin J Traumatol 2006;9(2):72–6.

[105] Nikolaou PK, Seaber AV, Glisson RR, et al. Anterior cruciate ligament allograft transplantation. Long-term function, histology, revascularization, and operative technique. Am J Sports Med 1986;14(5):348–60.

[106] Yamagishi T, Fujii K, Roppongi S, et al. Blood flow measurement in reconstructed anterior cruciate ligaments using laser Doppler flowmetry. Knee Surg Sports Traumatol Arthrosc 1998;6(3):160–4.

[107] Freedman KB, D'Amato MJ, Nedeff DD, et al. Arthroscopic anterior cruciate ligament reconstruction: a metaanalysis comparing patellar tendon and hamstring tendon autografts. Am J Sports Med 2003;31(1):2–11.

Peripheral Versus Aperture Fixation for Anterior Cruciate Ligament Reconstruction

Michael J. Elliott, MD[a,b,*], Christopher A. Kurtz, MD[b,c]

[a]Department of Orthopedics, Specialty Medical Group, Children's Hospital Central California, 9300 Valley Children's Place, Madera, California, CA 93636, USA
[b]Department of Orthopedics, Uniformed Services University of the Health Sciences, 4301 Jones Bridge Road, Bethesda, MD 20814, USA
[c]Division of Sports Medicine, Department of Orthopaedic Surgery, Naval Medical Center Portsmouth, 620 John Paul Jones Circle, Portsmouth Virginia, VA 23708, USA

Because both the young and the aging populations show an increasing interest in sports participation, the number of sports-related injuries, including injuries to knee ligaments, also seems to be increasing. Injuries to the anterior cruciate ligament (ACL) are more common than injuries to the other ligaments of the knee [1]. Clinical results show that nonoperative treatment of ACL injuries can result in poor functional outcomes [2–4]. In contrast, extra-articular ligaments, such as the medial collateral ligament, have shown excellent functional recovery after conservative treatment [5]. Injuries to extra-articular ligaments produce a hematoma that organizes into a fibrinogen mesh and collects inflammatory cells. This inflammatory cascade produces mediators that attract fibroblasts to the injured ligament. These cells then reorganize the granulation tissue to form scar or fibrous tissue. In the intra-articular ligament injury, the organization of a hematoma is limited by the presence of synovial fluid. Because of the poor results with conservative management, much energy and time has been focused on reconstructing the ACL so individuals may continue to participate in sporting activities.

Numerous mechanical and biologic factors must be considered to obtain a successful outcome of these complex ligament reconstructions. Of all factors

The views expressed in this article are those of the authors and do not reflect the official policy or position of the Department of the Navy, Department of Defense, or the United States Government.

KAC is a military service member (or employee of the U.S. Government). This work was prepared as part of his official duties. Title 17 U.S.C. 105 provides that "Copyright protection under this title is not available for any work of the United States Government." Title 17 U.S.C. 101 defines a United States Government work as a work prepared by a military service member or employee of the United States Government as part of that person's official duties.

*Corresponding author. E-mail address: melliott@childrenscentralcal.org (M.J. Elliott).

0278-5919/07/$ – see front matter
doi:10.1016/j.csm.2007.06.002

needed for a successful reconstruction, graft fixation has been a primary concern, as illustrated by the volumes of research produced on this topic [6–18]. During the last decade there has been a move toward rapid mobilization and rehabilitation of these patients. Rehabilitation protocols now emphasize immediate full range of motion, proprioception, and return of neuromuscular function allowing immediate weight bearing [19–21]. Graft fixation must be strong enough to permit early motion and weight bearing while still allowing biologic incorporation of the graft without loss of stability. Numerous fixation methods have been used to provide stability while allowing graft incorporation into the bone tunnels [6,10,11,13,18,22–40]. This article explores and reviews the concepts of fixation location and how they affect ultimate outcomes of these reconstructive procedures.

ANTERIOR CRUCIATE LIGAMENT ANATOMY

The anatomy of the native ACL becomes important when performing a reconstruction. Knowledge of native anatomy allows precise graft placement. The ACL consists of two main bundles–anterolateral and posteromedial–and is the primary restraint to anterior translation of the tibia [41,42]. The ACL inserts on the tibial plateau medial to the insertion of he anterior horn of the lateral meniscus [42–44]. The femoral attachment is on the posterior aspect of the medial surface of the lateral femoral condyle. The attachment site forms a semicircle with a straight anterior border and a convex posterior portion. It is these attachment points that have spawned controversy as to which fixation location allows the performance of the graft to resemble most closely the performance of native ligament it has been designed to replace. It is proposed that fixation at the precise origin and insertion of the native ACL aperture fixation results in a stronger and more functional reconstruction. In contrast, fixation away from these anatomic sites at the cortical bone peripheral fixation may result in inferior fixation.

BIOMECHANICS

Because of the poor ability of the native ACL to heal, primary repair has given way to the use of grafts for reconstruction. The most common grafts used today are the bone-patellar tendon-bone (BPTB) [23,45–53], the quadrupled semitendinosus/gracilis (hamstring) tendon graft, and various allografts [14,19,54–66]. Each tendon graft has unique properties, advantages, and disadvantages. As such, multiple fixation options have evolved based on graft type. Numerous studies have analyzed these different fixation options. The goal is to approximate the strength and functionality of the native ACL. In general, all graft options can approach or exceed the strength of the native ACL; fixation can be the weak link. Graft fixation must be strong enough to support the stress of daily activities and the stress of accelerated rehabilitation, while also allowing maximal incorporation of the graft into bone. Both aperture- and peripheral-based fixation devices have been used with varying degrees of success. Peripheral fixation devices secure the graft at a point distal to the origin or insertion of the native graft (Fig. 1). Examples include the

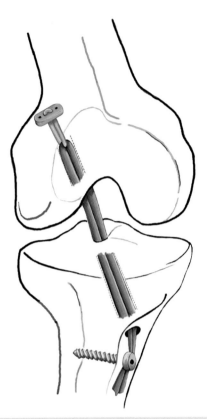

Fig. 1. Peripheral fixation on femur and tibia.

EndoButton (Smith & Nephew, Warsaw, Indiana), polyester buttons, staples, and suture posts. Central fixation that is still distal to the aperture is accomplished with interference screws and cross-pin devices (Fig. 2). True aperture fixation at both origin and insertion requires the use of soft tissue devices that fix the graft at the tunnel entrances (Fig. 3). These various reconstruction techniques, fixation devices, and graft types have an important impact on the biomechanical properties of the reconstruction. Much of the existing data on these biomechanical properties is based on tests looking at single load-to-failure [26,29,56,67,68]. Although many fixation devices provide strength that is equal to or greater than the ultimate strength of the native ACL, motion between the graft and bone is thought to provide an overall weaker reconstruction. This motion of the ACL graft in the tunnels has been proposed as a cause for tunnel widening [18,69,70]. Enlargement of the femoral and tibial tunnels after ACL reconstruction with both BPTB and hamstring grafts has been noted on radiographs [69–75]. It is hypothesized that peripheral fixation (away from the origin and insertion of the native graft site) results in more tunnel widening than seen with aperture fixation (at the point of origin and insertion).

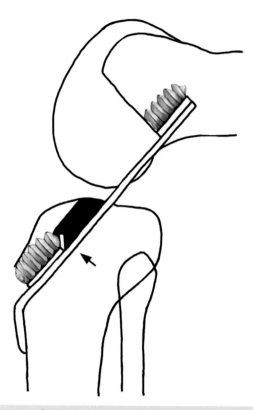

Fig. 2. Central fixation at the tibial screw. Arrow indicates fixation point in central portion of the tibial tunnel.

Therefore, to optimize fixation and reduce graft motion, it has been proposed that securing the graft at the origin and insertion of the native ACL provides superior fixation and eventually better clinical results. Although peripheral fixation has a long and successful track record, there have been problems with tunnel widening caused by creep of the graft because of an inherent weakness in the linkage system. Therefore aperture fixation has been hypothesized to be superior. To investigate how fixation position affects the property of the graft, Ishibashi and colleagues [76] used a robotic testing system to study cadaveric knees. Utilizing a BPTB graft, fixation was placed sequentially at three different locations: proximal (aperture), central, and distal (peripheral). The investigators found that the proximal fixation provided the most stable knee with the least amount of translation and rotation.

Another concern with peripheral fixation has been creep. Peripheral fixation allows more graft creep and subsequent weakening of the bone–tendon interface. Grover and colleagues [77] tested the concept of graft creep to see if there was a linear relationship between creep in a graft and increased knee laxity. In their study, cadaveric knees were reconstructed with the fixation

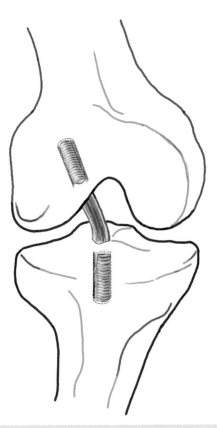

Fig. 3. Aperture fixation on femur and tibia. Screws at the tunnel entrance into the joint.

changed sequentially to represent an increase in graft length from 1 to 5 mm. They found a liner relationship in which the amount of graft creep translated directly to knee laxity [77]. In a separate study by Coleridge and Amis [32] evaluating graft creep in association with tibial fixation; cadaveric human tibias were fixed with various types of fixation, both peripheral and central. In this study, no device demonstrated any graft creep on cyclic testing; however, all devices were a variant of direct fixation, and none had any suture linkage [32]. To determine if there was any difference between peripheral and aperture fixation in the femur, Brown and colleagues [78] tested various fixation techniques on cadaver knees. Once fixed, the ACL complex was cyclically loaded, and an analysis of graft motion was performed. These same grafts also were tested to failure. Investigators found that there was little motion difference between peripheral and aperture fixation except when suture linkage was used as part of the fixation construct.

Two additional studies have compared peripheral and aperture fixation [79,80]. One study used porcine femurs; the other used human cadaver knees.

Both demonstrated that fixation at the aperture of the tunnel provided greater graft stiffness and greater pull-out strength. Although not specifically testing peripheral or aperture fixation, Milano and colleagues [16] tested fixation that relied on cancellous versus corticocancellous fixation. They found that screws in the cancellous bone allowed more slippage than peripheral corticalcancellous fixation devices. Scheffler and colleagues [59] demonstrated that anatomic direct screw fixation produced the best structural properties, but graft slippage was still present when soft tissue interference screws were used. They concluded that fixation might be improved by using a hybrid fixation system. Although the biomechanical literature seems to favor aperture fixation, it still is unknown if the functional outcomes of aperture fixation will be better than those achieved with peripheral fixation.

CLINICAL RESULTS

Biomechanically, aperture fixation produces a stiffer graft with less creep. In addition, peripherally fixed grafts may result in tunnel widening [73,81,82]. It remains to be seen, however, if these observations translate into clinical significance. Tunnel widening is associated with peripheral graft fixation. In one randomized, prospective study [81], both hamstring and BPTB grafts were fixed with peripheral EndoButton fixation. Both groups developed tunnel widening on follow-up radiographs. Although the hamstring group showed slightly wider tunnels, clinical outcomes with both types of grafts were excellent, with no correlation between tunnel widening and clinical results. If tunnel expansion is caused by ligament laxity, as hypothesized by Grover and colleagues [77], patients who have tunnel widening should have increased laxity. Simonian and colleagues [57], however, found that grafts fixed with peripheral fixation did indeed develop expansion of the bone tunnel, but this expansion did not translate into laxity. In short, although these techniques do result in motion that creates tunnel dilatation, the observed changes have not been associated clinically with laxity.

Does aperture fixation decrease tunnel widening and does it translate into a more stable knee? Barber and colleagues [83] compared two groups of BPTB reconstructions, one with standard screws placed more peripherally and one with screws placed at the aperture of the tunnels. They found that 90% of the peripherally fixed grafts demonstrated a 2-mm increase in tunnel diameter. In the aperture group, there was no increase in the tunnel width. Despite these radiographic differences, there was no clinical difference between the groups in relation to Lysholm, Tegner, International Knee Documentation Committee activity levels, KT-1000 (MEDmetric Corporation, San Diego, California), and physical examination parameters. In hamstring ACL reconstruction, both peripheral fixation and aperture fixation have produced stable knees. A prospective study looking at these fixation techniques found tunnel widening in both groups but stability on clinical examination [66]. It is possible that widening of the tunnels in the aperture group could have resulted from the cancellous fixation. Graft motion has been demonstrated biomechanically with cancellous fixation techniques [84]. Other clinical studies have compared peripheral and aperture fixation with much the same results [66,81,85–87]. Tunnel widening was greater with peripheral peripheral than with aperture fixation. The final outcome has been consistent in all these studies: although peripheral fixation does result in tunnel widening, the clinical outcomes are the same between fixation groups.

SUMMARY

Aperture fixation is appealing because it is an attempt to recreate the native ACL fixation points. Biomechanically, fixation at the graft tunnel origin provides a stiffer construct with less chance of graft motion in the tunnels. In addition, in the clinical setting aperture fixation has been shown to decrease graft tunnel widening after rehabilitation. Although theoretically aperture fixation should be a superior fixation technique, the functional outcomes have shown no difference between fixation techniques. One demonstrated benefit of aperture fixation is the decrease in graft tunnel expansion. Although this reduction has not affected clinical outcomes, it may be important when grafts fail and revision surgery is required. Combining the strength of peripheral fixation with the more anatomic position of aperture fixation might produce a clinically more stable knee. To determine if aperture fixation truly can provide a more stable knee with a better clinical outcome will require a large, randomized study with long-term outcomes.

References

[1] Majewski M, Susanne H, Klaus S. Epidemiology of athletic knee injuries: a 10-year study. Knee 2006;13(3):184–8.

[2] Drongowski RA, Coran AG, Wojtys EM. Predictive value of meniscal and chondral injuries in conservatively treated anterior cruciate ligament injuries. Arthroscopy 1994;10(1): 97–102.

[3] Kannus P, Jarvinen M. Conservatively treated tears of the anterior cruciate ligament. Long-term results. J Bone Joint Surg Am 1987;69(7):1007–12.

[4] Neusel E, Maibaum S, Rompe G. Five-year results of conservatively treated tears of the anterior cruciate ligament. Arch Orthop Trauma Surg 1996;115(6):332–6.

[5] Ballmer PM, Jakob RP. The non operative treatment of isolated complete tears of the medial collateral ligament of the knee. A prospective study. Arch Orthop Trauma Surg 1988; 107(5):273–6.

[6] Butler JC, Branch TP, Hutton WC. Optimal graft fixation—the effect of gap size and screw size on bone plug fixation in ACL reconstruction. Arthroscopy 1994;10(5):524–9.

[7] Beynnon BD, Uh BS, Pyne JI, et al. Semitendinosus and gracilis tendon graft fixation for ACL reconstructions. Iowa Orthop J 1996;16:118–21.

[8] Williams A, Myers PT. Quality of tibial fixation in ACL reconstructions. Am J Sports Med 1997;25(3):417–8.

[9] Cuppone M, Seedhom BB. Effect of implant lengthening and mode of fixation on knee laxity after ACL reconstruction with an artificial ligament: a cadaveric study. J Orthop Sci 2001;6(3):253–61.

[10] Klein SA, Nyland J, Kocabey Y, et al. Tendon graft fixation in ACL reconstruction: in vitro evaluation of bioabsorbable tenodesis screw. Acta Orthop Scand 2004;75(1):84–8.

[11] Berg TL, Paulos LE. Endoscopic ACL reconstruction using Stryker Biosteon cross-pin femoral fixation and interlock cross-pin tibial fixation. Surg Technol Int 2004;12:239–44.

[12] Hertel P, Behrend H, Cierpinski T, et al. ACL reconstruction using bone-patellar tendon-bone press-fit fixation: 10-year clinical results. Knee Surg Sports Traumatol Arthrosc 2005;13(4): 248–55.

[13] Singhal MC, Fites BS, Johnson DL. Fixation devices in ACL surgery: what do I need to know? Orthopedics 2005;28(9):920–4.

[14] Rose T, Hepp P, Venus J, et al. Prospective randomized clinical comparison of femoral transfixation versus bioscrew fixation in hamstring tendon ACL reconstruction—a preliminary report. Knee Surg Sports Traumatol Arthrosc 2006;14(8):730–8.

[15] Harilainen A, Linko E, Sandelin J. Randomized prospective study of ACL reconstruction with interference screw fixation in patellar tendon autografts versus femoral metal plate suspension and tibial post fixation in hamstring tendon autografts: 5-year clinical and radiological follow-up results. Knee Surg Sports Traumatol Arthrosc 2006;14(6):517–28.

[16] Milano G, Mulas PD, Ziranu F, et al. Comparison between different femoral fixation devices for ACL reconstruction with doubled hamstring tendon graft: a biomechanical analysis. Arthroscopy 2006;22(6):660–8.

[17] Weimann A, Zantop T, Herbort M, et al. Initial fixation strength of a hybrid technique for femoral ACL graft fixation. Knee Surg Sports Traumatol Arthrosc 2006;14(11):1122–9.

[18] Brand J Jr, Weiler A, Caborn DN, et al. Graft fixation in cruciate ligament reconstruction. Am J Sports Med 2000;28(5):761–74.

[19] Vadala A, Iorio R, De Carli A, et al. The effect of accelerated, brace free, rehabilitation on bone tunnel enlargement after ACL reconstruction using hamstring tendons: a CT study. Knee Surg Sports Traumatol Arthrosc 2007;15(4):365–71.

[20] Bollen SR. BASK instructional lecture 3: rehabilitation after ACL reconstruction. Knee 2001;8(1):75–7.

[21] Shelbourne KD, Klotz C. What I have learned about the ACL: utilizing a progressive rehabilitation scheme to achieve total knee symmetry after anterior cruciate ligament reconstruction. J Orthop Sci 2006;11(3):318–25.

[22] Abate JA, Fadale PD, Hulstyn MJ, et al. Initial fixation strength of polylactic acid interference screws in anterior cruciate ligament reconstruction. Arthroscopy 1998;14(3):278–84.

[23] Al-Husseiny M, Batterjee K. Press-fit fixation in reconstruction of anterior cruciate ligament, using bone-patellar tendon-bone graft. Knee Surg Sports Traumatol Arthrosc 2004;12(2): 104–9.

[24] Arneja S, Froese W, MacDonald P. Augmentation of femoral fixation in hamstring anterior cruciate ligament reconstruction with a bioabsorbable bead: a prospective single-blind randomized clinical trial. Am J Sports Med 2004;32(1):159–63.

[25] Au AG, Otto DD, Raso VJ, et al. Investigation of a hybrid method of soft tissue graft fixation for anterior cruciate ligament reconstruction. Knee 2005;12(2):149–53.

[26] Aune AK, Ekeland A, Cawley PW. Interference screw fixation of hamstring vs patellar tendon grafts for anterior cruciate ligament reconstruction. Knee Surg Sports Traumatol Arthrosc 1998;6(2):99–102.

[27] Black KP, Saunders MM. Expansion anchors for use in anterior cruciate ligament (ACL) reconstruction: establishing proof of concept in a benchtop analysis. Med Eng Phys 2005;27(5):425–34.

[28] Bryan JM, Bach BR Jr, Bush-Joseph CA, et al. Comparison of "inside-out" and "outside-in" interference screw fixation for anterior cruciate ligament surgery in a bovine knee. Arthroscopy 1996;12(1):76–81.

[29] Caborn DN, Urban WP Jr, Johnson DL, et al. Biomechanical comparison between bioscrew and titanium alloy interference screws for bone-patellar tendon-bone graft fixation in anterior cruciate ligament reconstruction. Arthroscopy 1997;13(2):229–32.

[30] Chandratreya AP, Aldridge MJ. Top tips for RIGIDfix femoral fixation. Arthroscopy 2004;20(6):e59–61.

[31] Clark R, Olsen RE, Larson BJ, et al. Cross-pin femoral fixation: a new technique for hamstring anterior cruciate ligament reconstruction of the knee. Arthroscopy 1998;14(3):258–67.

[32] Coleridge SD, Amis AA. A comparison of five tibial-fixation systems in hamstring-graft anterior cruciate ligament reconstruction. Knee Surg Sports Traumatol Arthrosc 2004;12(5): 391–7.

[33] Fink C, Benedetto KP, Hackl W, et al. Bioabsorbable polyglyconate interference screw fixation in anterior cruciate ligament reconstruction: a prospective computed tomography-controlled study. Arthroscopy 2000;16(5):491–8.

[34] Gobbi A, Mahajan S, Tuy B, et al. Hamstring graft tibial fixation: biomechanical properties of different linkage systems. Knee Surg Sports Traumatol Arthrosc 2002;10(6):330–4.

[35] Hantes ME, Dailiana Z, Zachos VC, et al. Anterior cruciate ligament reconstruction using the bio-transfix femoral fixation device and anteromedial portal technique. Knee Surg Sports Traumatol Arthrosc 2006;14(5):497–501.

[36] Harilainen A, Sandelin J, Jansson KA. Cross-pin femoral fixation versus metal interference screw fixation in anterior cruciate ligament reconstruction with hamstring tendons: results of a controlled prospective randomized study with 2-year follow-up. Arthroscopy 2005;21(1):25–33.

[37] Kocabey Y, Nawab A, Caborn DN, et al. EndoPearl augmentation of bioabsorbable interference screw fixation of a soft tissue tendon graft in a tibial tunnel. Arthroscopy 2004;20(6):658–61.

[38] Mariani PP, Camillieri G, Margheritini F. Transcondylar screw fixation in anterior cruciate ligament reconstruction. Arthroscopy 2001;17(7):717–23.

[39] Novak PJ, Wexler GM, Williams JS Jr, et al. Comparison of screw post fixation and free bone block interference fixation for anterior cruciate ligament soft tissue grafts: biomechanical considerations. Arthroscopy 1996;12(4):470–3.

[40] Zysk SP, Kruger A, Baur A, et al. Tripled semitendinosus anterior cruciate ligament reconstruction with Endobutton fixation: a 2-3-year follow-up study of 35 patients. Acta Orthop Scand 2000;71(4):381–6.

[41] Butler DL, Noyes FR, Grood ES. Ligamentous restraints to anterior-posterior drawer in the human knee. A biomechanical study. J Bone Joint Surg Am 1980;62(2):259–70.

[42] Arnoczky SP. Anatomy of the anterior cruciate ligament. Clin Orthop Relat Res 1983;172: 19–25.

[43] Morgan CD, Kalman VR, Grawl DM. Definitive landmarks for reproducible tibial tunnel placement in anterior cruciate ligament reconstruction. Arthroscopy 1995;11(3):275–88.

[44] Girgis FG, Marshall JL, Monajem A. The cruciate ligaments of the knee joint. Anatomical, functional and experimental analysis. Clin Orthop Relat Res 1975;106:216–31.

[45] Rubinstein RA Jr, Shelbourne KD, VanMeter CD, et al. Isolated autogenous bone-patellar tendon-bone graft site morbidity. Am J Sports Med 1994;22(3):324–7.

[46] Shelbourne KD, Patel DV. ACL reconstruction using the autogenous bone-patellar tendon-bone graft: open two-incision technique. Instr Course Lect 1996;45:245–52.

[47] Mariani PP, Adriani E, Santori N, et al. Arthroscopic posterior cruciate ligament reconstruction with bone-tendon-bone patellar graft. Knee Surg Sports Traumatol Arthrosc 1997; 5(4):239–44.

[48] Auge WK 2nd, Yifan K. A technique for resolution of graft-tunnel length mismatch in central third bone-patellar tendon-bone anterior cruciate ligament reconstruction. Arthroscopy 1999;15(8):877–81.

[49] Shelbourne KD, O'Shea JJ. Revision anterior cruciate ligament reconstruction using the contralateral bone-patellar tendon-bone graft. Instr Course Lect 2002;51:343–6.

[50] Paessler HH, Mastrokalos DS. Anterior cruciate ligament reconstruction using semitendinosus and gracilis tendons, bone patellar tendon, or quadriceps tendon-graft with press-fit fixation without hardware. A new and innovative procedure. Orthop Clin North Am 2003;34(1):49–64.

[51] Yasuda K, Tomita F, Yamazaki S, et al. The effect of growth factors on biomechanical properties of the bone-patellar tendon-bone graft after anterior cruciate ligament reconstruction: a canine model study. Am J Sports Med 2004;32(4):870–80.

[52] Tecklenburg K, Hoser C, Sailer R, et al. [ACL reconstruction with bone-patellar tendon-bone graft and proximal fixation with the EndoButton: a 2- to 5-year follow-up]. Unfallchirurg 2005;108(9):721–7 [in German].

[53] Sadovsky P, Musil D, Filip L, et al. Reconstruction of the anterior cruciate ligament: comparison of patellar bone-tendon-bone and hamstring tendon graft methods. Part 1. Evaluation of patients treated by the patellar bone-tendon-bone graft technique. Acta Chir Orthop Traumatol Cech 2005;72(4):235–8 [in Czech].

[54] Wilcox JF, Gross JA, Sibel R, et al. Anterior cruciate ligament reconstruction with hamstring tendons and cross-pin femoral fixation compared with patellar tendon autografts. Arthroscopy 2005;21(10):1186–92.

[55] Weimann A, Rodieck M, Zantop T, et al. Primary stability of hamstring graft fixation with biodegradable suspension versus interference screws. Arthroscopy 2005;21(3):266–74.

[56] Steiner ME, Hecker AT, Brown CH Jr, et al. Comparison of hamstring and patellar tendon grafts. Am J Sports Med. 1994;22(2):240–6 [discussion: 246–7].

[57] Simonian PT, Erickson MS, Larson RV, et al. Tunnel expansion after hamstring anterior cruciate ligament reconstruction with 1-incision EndoButton femoral fixation. Arthroscopy 2000;16(7):707–14.

[58] Shino K, Pflaster DS. Comparison of eccentric and concentric screw placement for hamstring graft fixation in the tibial tunnel. Knee Surg Sports Traumatol Arthrosc 2000;8(2):73–5.

[59] Scheffler SU, Sudkamp NP, Gockenjan A, et al. Biomechanical comparison of hamstring and patellar tendon graft anterior cruciate ligament reconstruction techniques: the impact of fixation level and fixation method under cyclic loading. Arthroscopy 2002;18(3): 304–15.

[60] Phillips BB, Cain EL, Dlabach JA, et al. Correlation of interference screw insertion torque with depth of placement in the tibial tunnel using a quadrupled semitendinosus-gracilis graft in anterior cruciate ligament reconstruction. Arthroscopy 2004;20(10):1026–9.

[61] Prodromos CC, Han YS, Keller BL, et al. Stability results of hamstring anterior cruciate ligament reconstruction at 2- to 8-year follow-up. Arthroscopy 2005;21(2):138–46.

[62] Robert H, Es-Sayeh J, Heymann D, et al. Hamstring insertion site healing after anterior cruciate ligament reconstruction in patients with symptomatic hardware or repeat rupture: a histologic study in 12 patients. Arthroscopy 2003;19(9):948–54.

[63] Kousa P, Jarvinen TL, Vihavainen M, et al. The fixation strength of six hamstring tendon graft fixation devices in anterior cruciate ligament reconstruction. Part II: tibial site. Am J Sports Med 2003;31(2):182–8.

[64] Laxdal G, Kartus J, Hansson L, et al. A prospective randomized comparison of bone-patellar tendon-bone and hamstring grafts for anterior cruciate ligament reconstruction. Arthroscopy 2005;21(1):34–42.

[65] Laxdal G, Sernert N, Ejerhed L, et al. A prospective comparison of bone-patellar tendon-bone and hamstring tendon grafts for anterior cruciate ligament reconstruction in male patients. Knee Surg Sports Traumatol Arthrosc 2007;15(2):115–25.

[66] Ma CB, Francis K, Towers J, et al. Hamstring anterior cruciate ligament reconstruction: a comparison of bioabsorbable interference screw and EndoButton-post fixation. Arthroscopy 2004;20(2):122–8.

[67] Weiler A, Windhagen HJ, Raschke MJ, et al. Biodegradable interference screw fixation exhibits pull-out force and stiffness similar to titanium screws. Am J Sports Med 1998;26(1):119–26.

[68] Rowden NJ, Sher D, Rogers GJ, et al. Anterior cruciate ligament graft fixation. Initial comparison of patellar tendon and semitendinosus autografts in young fresh cadavers. Am J Sports Med 1997;25(4):472–8.

[69] Clatworthy MG, Annear P, Bulow JU, et al. Tunnel widening in anterior cruciate ligament reconstruction: a prospective evaluation of hamstring and patella tendon grafts. Knee Surg Sports Traumatol Arthrosc 1999;7(3):138–45.

[70] Hoher J, Moller HD, Fu FH. Bone tunnel enlargement after anterior cruciate ligament reconstruction: fact or fiction? Knee Surg Sports Traumatol Arthrosc 1998;6(4): 231–40.

[71] Zijl JA, Kleipool AE, Willems WJ. Comparison of tibial tunnel enlargement after anterior cruciate ligament reconstruction using patellar tendon autograft or allograft. Am J Sports Med 2000;28(4):547–51.

[72] Peyrache MD, Djian P, Christel P, et al. Tibial tunnel enlargement after anterior cruciate ligament reconstruction by autogenous bone-patellar tendon-bone graft. Knee Surg Sports Traumatol Arthrosc 1996;4(1):2–8.

[73] Nebelung W, Becker R, Merkel M, et al. Bone tunnel enlargement after anterior cruciate ligament reconstruction with semitendinosus tendon using Endobutton fixation on the femoral side. Arthroscopy 1998;14(8):810–5.

[74] Jansson KA, Harilainen A, Sandelin J, et al. Bone tunnel enlargement after anterior cruciate ligament reconstruction with the hamstring autograft and endobutton fixation technique. A clinical, radiographic and magnetic resonance imaging study with 2 years follow-up. Knee Surg Sports Traumatol Arthrosc 1999;7(5):290–5.

[75] Fahey M, Indelicato PA. Bone tunnel enlargement after anterior cruciate ligament replacement. Am J Sports Med 1994;22(3):410–4.

[76] Ishibashi Y, Rudy TW, Livesay GA, et al. The effect of anterior cruciate ligament graft fixation site at the tibia on knee stability: evaluation using a robotic testing system. Arthroscopy 1997;13(2):177–82.

[77] Grover D, Thompson D, Hull ML, et al. Empirical relationship between lengthening an anterior cruciate ligament graft and increases in knee anterior laxity: a human cadaveric study. J Biomech Eng 2006;128(6):969–72.

[78] Brown CH Jr, Wilson DR, Hecker AT, et al. Graft-bone motion and tensile properties of hamstring and patellar tendon anterior cruciate ligament femoral graft fixation under cyclic loading. Arthroscopy 2004;20(9):922–35.

[79] Benfield D, Otto DD, Bagnall KM, et al. Stiffness characteristics of hamstring tendon graft fixation methods at the femoral site. Int Orthop 2005;29(1):35–8.

[80] Hayes DA, Watts MC, Tevelen GA, et al. Central versus peripheral tibial screw placement in hamstring anterior cruciate ligament reconstruction: in vitro biomechanics. Arthroscopy 2005;21(6):703–6.

[81] Webster KE, Feller JA, Hameister KA. Bone tunnel enlargement following anterior cruciate ligament reconstruction: a randomised comparison of hamstring and patellar tendon grafts with 2-year follow-up. Knee Surg Sports Traumatol Arthrosc 2001;9(2):86–91.

[82] Otsuka H, Ishibashi Y, Tsuda E, et al. Comparison of three techniques of anterior cruciate ligament reconstruction with bone-patellar tendon-bone graft. Differences in anterior tibial translation and tunnel enlargement with each technique. Am J Sports Med 2003;31(2): 282–8.

[83] Barber FA, Spruill B, Sheluga M. The effect of outlet fixation on tunnel widening. Arthroscopy 2003;19(5):485–92.

[84] Milano G, Mulas PD, Sanna-Passino E, et al. Evaluation of bone plug and soft tissue anterior cruciate ligament graft fixation over time using transverse femoral fixation in a sheep model. Arthroscopy 2005;21(5):532–9.

[85] Buelow JU, Siebold R, Ellermann A. A prospective evaluation of tunnel enlargement in anterior cruciate ligament reconstruction with hamstrings: extracortical versus anatomical fixation. Knee Surg Sports Traumatol Arthrosc 2002;10(2):80–5.

[86] Fauno P, Kaalund S. Tunnel widening after hamstring anterior cruciate ligament reconstruction is influenced by the type of graft fixation used: a prospective randomized study. Arthroscopy 2005;21(11):1337–41.

[87] Hersekli MA, Akpinar S, Ozalay M, et al. Tunnel enlargement after arthroscopic anterior cruciate ligament reconstruction: comparison of bone-patellar tendon-bone and hamstring autografts. Adv Ther 2004;21(2):123–31.

Biomechanics of Intratunnel Anterior Cruciate Ligament Graft Fixation

Neal C. Chen, MD[a,b,c], Jeff C. Brand, Jr, MD[d,*],
Charles H. Brown, Jr, MD[e]

[a]Combined Harvard Orthopaedic Residency Program, Boston, MA, USA
[b]Hand and Upper Extremity Service, Massachusetts General Hospital,
55 Fruit Street, Boston, MA 02114, USA
[c]Sports Medicine and Shoulder Service, Hospital for Special Surgery,
535 East 70th Street, New York, NY 10021, USA
[d]Alexandria Orthopaedics and Sports Medicine Asssociates, 1500 Irving, Alexandria,
MN 56308, USA
[e]Abu Dhabi Knee and Sports Medicine Centre, 6th Floor, Saif Tower, Electra Street,
P.O. Box 43330, Abu Dhabi, United Arab Emirates

I n 1983 Lambert [1] first introduced the technique of intratunnel anterior cruciate ligament (ACL) graft fixation by securing a vascularized bone-patellar tendon-bone ACL graft with 6.5-mm AO cancellous screws. Kurosaka and colleagues [2] demonstrated that fixation of a 10-mm bone-patellar tendon-bone ACL graft in human cadaveric knees with a custom-designed headless 9.0-mm fully threaded interference screw had better strength and stiffness than fixation with a 6.5-mm AO cancellous screw, staple fixation, or tying sutures over a button. Because of the many biomechanical studies demonstrating superior initial fixation properties and clinical outcomes studies demonstrating a high rate of success, interference screw fixation of bone-patellar tendon-bone grafts now is considered the standard against which all ACL graft-fixation techniques are compared [3,4]. Based on the success of interference screw fixation of bone-patellar tendon-bone ACL grafts, Pinczewski [5] in 1996 introduced the use of blunt, threaded metal interference screws to fix four-strand hamstring tendon ACL grafts, and in 1997 Fu [6] described quadrupled hamstring tendon grafts (QHTGs) for ACL reconstruction secured with a bioabsorbable interference screw.

Rigid initial graft fixation minimizes elongation and prevents failure at the graft-attachment sites, maintaining knee ligament stability during cyclical loading of the knee before biologic fixation of the ACL graft. The advantages of early joint motion, early weight bearing, and closed-chain exercises following ACL

---

*Corresponding author. E-mail address: bjbrand@info-link.net (J.C. Brand, Jr).

0278-5919/07/$ – see front matter
doi:10.1016/j.csm.2007.06.009

reconstruction have been well documented. These activities place greater demands on initial ACL graft fixation. One of the still unanswered questions regarding ACL graft fixation is, "How strong and stiff do the initial graft-fixation methods need to be to allow use of an accelerated ACL rehabilitation program?"

In the late 1960s Morrison [7,8], using force plate and gait analysis, estimated that the forces experienced by the ACL during activities of daily living ranged from 27 newtons (N) to 445 N. Noyes and colleagues [9] estimated that the ACL is loaded to approximately 454 N during activities of daily living. In vitro mechanical studies have demonstrated that the initial strength and stiffness of bone-patellar tendon-bone grafts and QHTGs far exceed the estimated loads on the ACL [9–11]. The forces placed on the ACL with rehabilitation exercises performed in the early postoperative period or during activities of daily living are unknown. The initial tensile properties of all current ACL graft-fixation methods are inferior to those of the ACL grafts themselves [12]. Therefore, the mechanical fixation of the ACL graft in the bone tunnels is the weak link in the early postoperative period.

This article discusses some of the limitations of in vitro biomechanical studies and reviews variables that influence the tensile properties of intratunnel fixation methods for bone-tendon-bone and soft tissue grafts.

LIMITATIONS OF BIOMECHANICAL STUDIES

Although in vitro biomechanical studies most commonly are used to evaluate initial ACL graft-fixation properties [13,14], these investigations have inherent limitations. First, the differing research models and biomechanical testing protocols make it difficult to compare the results of one study with those of another. Ideally, young human specimens are used for biomechanical testing; but the material properties of cortical and cancellous bone and of tendons and ligaments can vary greatly from specimen to specimen. Because of the lack of availability of human cadaveric specimens in the age range of patients typically undergoing ACL reconstruction, specimens from older donors often are used, or the same specimen is tested multiple times. Brown and colleagues [15] evaluated the initial fixation strength of bone-patellar tendon-bone grafts fixed with metal interference screws in the distal femur of bovine cadavers, of young human cadavers (mean age, 41 years; range. 33–52 years), and of elderly human cadavers (mean age, 73 years; range, 68–81 years). There was no significant difference in the failure load of the bovine (799 $\pm$ 261 N) and young human specimens (655 $\pm$ 186 N); however, the failure load of the elderly human specimens (382 $\pm$ 118 N) was significantly lower than that of the young human and bovine specimens. The authors concluded that elderly human cadavers are not appropriate models for ACL reconstruction fixation studies. Beynnon and Amis [13] have suggested testing male specimens below 65 years of age and female specimens below 50 years of age to minimize this problem. Performing multiple tests in the same specimen introduces carry-over effects that may affect the fixation properties of subsequent techniques tested after the first fixation method has been tested.

Animal models have the advantages of eliminating the potential variability introduced because of the large differences in bone mineral density (BMD) that exists in human specimens, and their availability eliminates the need to perform multiple tests using the same specimen. Because human and animal specimens differ in BMD and in the tensile properties of bone, the results of biomechanical tests performed using animal models cannot be compared directly with studies performed using human specimens. Aerssens and colleagues [16] have shown that human female femoral specimens (age range, 30–60 years) demonstrate lower BMD and failure stress than specimens from dogs, pigs, cows, or sheep. In this study the pig femur came closest to matching the BMD and failure stress of the human femur. Nagarkatti and colleagues [17] found significantly greater load to failure with both central quadriceps tendon and QHTG in porcine tibia tunnels (mean BMD, 1.42 g/cm^2) than in cadavers (mean age, 71 years; mean BMD, 0.30 g/cm^2) with an 8-mm bioabsorbable interference screw in a single load-to-failure test. Nurmi and colleagues [18] found a significant difference in bone mineral density of porcine tibias (210 $\pm$ 45 mg/cm^3) compared with those from young women (129 $\pm$ 30 mg/cm^3) and young men (134 $\pm$ 34 mg/cm^3). Because of the higher BMD and tensile properties of animal specimens, biomechanical tests performed in animal models tend to overestimate initial fixation properties (Table 1) [19–21]. This overestimation is particularly true for devices such as interference screws and cross-pins that rely on cancellous bone for fixation strength.

The in vitro biomechanical studies fail to account for the progressive healing of the ACL graft to the bone tunnel walls, which shifts the weak link from the ACL graft fixation–bone tunnel interface to the bone–ligament interface and eventually to the intra-articular part of the ACL graft [22]. Although the healing response does not affect graft-fixation properties in the early postoperative period, bony or soft tissue healing in the bone tunnels alters graft-fixation properties over time. There are few studies documenting the time frame for healing to occur at the ACL graft-fixation sites. Based on the studies of Clancy and colleagues [22] and Walton [23], the bone blocks of bone-tendon-bone grafts seem to heal to the bone tunnel wall by 6 weeks. In a dog model, Rodeo and colleagues [24] demonstrated the formation of Sharpey's fibers connecting the periphery of a soft tissue graft to the bone tunnel wall at 6 weeks. Mechanical fixation was not achieved until 12 weeks, however. In a sheep model with transverse femoral fixation, bone plug fixation was stronger than graft strength at 1 month after implantation, whereas soft tissue tendon incorporation was weaker than the graft until 2 months [25]. Soft tissue grafts take longer than bone-tendon-bone grafts to re-establish mechanical strength at the graft–tunnel interface.

Two types of biomechanical tests are used commonly to evaluate the mechanical behavior of ACL ligament-fixation techniques [13,14]. Single-cycle load-to-failure tests, the most prevalent, attempt to simulate the response of the graft-fixation technique to a sudden mechanical overload event such as a slip or fall. The load–displacement curve can be analyzed to determine the ultimate failure load, yield load, linear stiffness, and displacement at failure.

Table 1
Biomechanical studies with similar methodology that tested bone-patella tendon-bone grafts in a bone tunnel fixed with an interference screw[a]

Construct[b]	Substrate[c]	Failure (N)[d]	Failure Mode[e]
9 × 20-mm metal interference screw, endoscopic on the femur [19]	Bovine	1198 (93)	Bone plug site: failure of interference screw fit fixation or ligament avulsion
7 × 20-mm metal interference screw, endoscopic on the femur [19]	Bovine	1161 (93)	Bone plug site: failure of interference screw fit fixation or ligament avulsion
7 × 25-mm bioabsorbable interference screw, endoscopic [20]	Bovine	1151 (472)	Bone-screw interface, interligamentous failures[f]
7 × 25-mm bioabsorbable interference screw, outside-in [20]	Bovine	1017 (409)	Bone-screw interface, interligamentous failures
7 × 20-mm metal interference screw, outside-in [21]	Bovine	768.4 (163.3)	Attachment site failure or midsubstance ligament failure
9 × 20-mm metal interference screw, outside-in [21]	Bovine	728.2 (252.6)	Attachment site failure or midsubstance ligament failure
7 × 20-mm metal interference screw, endoscopic in either 0 or 10° of divergence [38]	Porcine	607 (46)	Not reported
7 × 25-mm metal interference screw, endoscopic [3]	Human (mean age, 69.5 years)	588 (282)	Bone plug fractured, femoral screw pullout, bone tendon rupture
9 × 20-mm bioabsorbable interference screw, outside-in [46]	Bovine	564.5 (272.3)	Bone plug pullout on the tibial side
9 × 25-mm metal interference screw [3]	Human (mean age, 69.5 years)	423 (175)	Pullout around the femoral or tibial screw
Interference screw, endoscopic [30]	Human (mean age, 79 years)	256 (130)	Bone block pullout, bone block fracture
Interference screw, outside-in [30]	Human (mean age, 79 years)	235 (124)	Bone block pullout, bone block fracture

[a]This table demonstrates that the maximum failure loads of bovine and porcine specimens exceed those of many human specimens.
[b]Construct describes the type of interference screw and the manner of insertion.
[c]Substrate is the type of bone that was used in the investigation.
[d]Failure is the maximum load at failure in Newtons (N).
[e]Failure mode describes the type of failure observed at the maximum failure load. The studies are listed in order of descending maximum load at failure.
[f]Interligamentous or midsubstance failures of the graft are rare in human studies because the maximum load at failure of the graft-fixation construct is below that of the ligament.

Single load-to-failure testing identifies the weak link in the fixation system. The mode and site of the fixation failure is well defined, and an upper limit of the strength of the graft-fixation construct is established. Because failure testing attempts to replicate traumatic loading conditions, a high rate of elongation (typically 100%/s) is used.

The second testing method is cyclic loading of the bone–ACL graft-fixation complex that evaluates the resistance to elongation or slippage under repetitive submaximal failure loads over time. Cyclic testing attempts to approximate the loading conditions associated with rehabilitation exercises or activities of daily living in the early postoperative period before biologic fixation of the graft. A load-control test often is performed with the upper and lower loads controlled, and the displacement of the ACL graft relative to the bone is measured. The difference in the distance between markers on the bone and ACL graft at the beginning and the end of the test represents the elongation or slippage of the ACL graft with respect to the bone. Unfortunately, there is little agreement on the force limits or the number of cycles that should be performed, making it difficult to compare data from one study to another. Beynnon and Amis [13] have recommended force limits between 150 N and −150 N and 1000 load cycles. One thousand cycles approximates 1 week of flexion-extension loading of the knee [14]. The number of cycles is limited by technical issues, such as keeping the specimen moist during testing and the thawing of the freeze clamps that grip soft tissue ACL grafts.

Despite these limitations, in vitro biomechanical laboratory testing can provide useful information on the performance of ACL ligament-fixation techniques. In summary, single load-to-failure testing evaluates the initial strength and stiffness of the bone–ACL graft-fixation complex, and cyclic testing provides information on slippage and progressive elongation at the graft fixation sites that occur as a result of rehabilitation exercises or activities of daily living in the early postoperative period before biologic healing has occurred.

BONE MINERAL DENSITY

Because intratunnel fixation methods depend on the graft-fixation device generating friction between the bone tunnel wall and the ACL replacement graft, BMD is an important variable influencing initial fixation strength and stiffness and resistance to slippage during cyclic loading. In humans BMD decreases with age, and the BMD of females is less than that of males. Cassim and colleagues [26] found that the fixation strength of bone-patellar tendon-bone grafts fixed with metal interference screws in human specimens with a mean age of 79 years resulted in a 42% decrease in failure load compared with specimens with a mean age of 35 years. The BMD of the proximal tibia is significantly lower than that of the distal femur [27]. Tibial fixation devices must resist shear forces applied parallel to the axis of the tibial bone tunnel that has a lower BMD. For these reasons, tibial fixation is the weak link in ACL graft fixation.

Although BMD is a critical factor, there are other variables that correlate with initial fixation properties. In a bone-patella tendon-bone model, Brown and colleagues [15] found that insertion torque, an indirect measure of BMD, was correlated linearly with pull-out force but with weak significance. Using elderly human cadaveric knees, Brand and colleagues [27] found that BMD measured using dual-energy X-ray absorptiometry and screw insertion torque explained 77% of the ultimate failure load observed in QHTG fixed with bioabsorbable interference screws in the distal femur and proximal tibia of human specimens. The R^2 value for the relationship between ultimate failure load and BMD was 0.65, indicating that BMD explained 65% of the ultimate failure load. This study found that a BMD of 0.6 g/cm^2 or higher resulted in better initial fixation properties. Using the proximal tibia of human cadaveric specimens (mean age, 40 ± 11 years; range, 17–54 years) and doubled tibialis tendons fixed with a tapered bioabsorbable screw, Jarvinen and colleagues [28] found that insertion torque was linearly correlated to fixation strength ($R^2 = 0.54$) and in their study was the variable most strongly predictive of fixation strength. Unfortunately, despite the correlation, insertion torque was a poor predictor of cyclic loading failure or single load-to-failure. The remainder of this article is aimed toward explicating the role and importance of secondary factors that influence the biomechanical properties of intratunnel graft fixation.

BONE-PATELLA TENDON-BONE FIXATION

The fixation properties of interference screw fixation of bone-tendon-bone grafts depend on the generation of friction generated by compression of the bone block into the bone tunnel wall and engagement of the interference screw threads. As illustrated in Fig. 1, factors that influence the initial tensile properties of interference screw fixation of bone-tendon-bone ACL grafts include

1. Screw diameter
2. Gap size
3. Screw length
4. Screw divergence

There is overlap between the effects of screw diameter and gap size on initial fixation properties. Kohn and Rose [29], using human cadaveric knees (mean age, 30 years), reported that tibial fixation using 9-mm screws was significantly stronger than tibial fixation using 7-mm screws. Based on their findings, they recommended against the using 7-mm screws for tibial fixation. With elderly human cadaveric specimens, two groups found no significant difference in the fixation strength of bone-patellar tendon-bone grafts fixed in the distal femur using retrograde or endoscopically inserted 7-mm screws and 9-mm screws inserted using a rear-entry or an antegrade technique [15,30]. The influence of screw diameter on initial fixation properties is probably most relevant when there is a significant size discrepancy between the bone block and the bone tunnel wall; this difference often is referred to as "gap size."

After studying various fixation methods, Kurosaka and colleagues [2] hypothesized that the gap size between the bone block and bone tunnel was a critical factor in interference screw fixation. Butler and colleagues [31], in

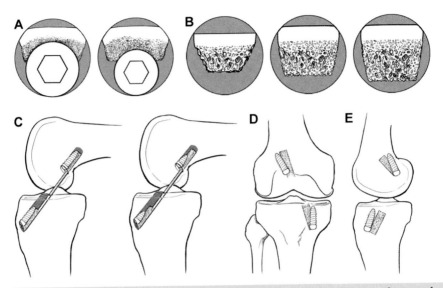

Fig. 1. Factors that influence the initial tensile properties of interference screw fixation of bone-tendon-bone ACL grafts. (*A*) Screw diameter: effect of a larger screw on bone plug. (*B*) Gap size: increase in gap size decreases strength of construct. (*C*) Screw length: lateral view of graft with longer (*left panel*) and shorter (*right panel*) interference screws. In bone-tendon-bone grafts screw length does not affect screw pullout significantly. (*D*) Screw divergence: anteroposterior view of the knee showing screw divergence from the tunnel. (*E*) Screw divergence, lateral view.

a porcine study, found that, with a gap size of 3 to 4 mm, increasing the screw diameter size from 7 mm to 9 mm significantly increased the load at which failure occurred. With a similar porcine experimental model, Reznik and colleagues [32] demonstrated that gap size significantly influenced the ultimate failure load of bone-tendon-bone grafts fixed in 10-mm bone tunnels with 7-mm screws. When the gap between the bone block and bone tunnel wall was 4 mm or more, increasing the screw diameter to 9 mm increased the failure load by 97%. When the gap was larger than 4 mm and a 9-mm screw was used, however, the results were inferior to using a 7-mm screw with a gap of less than 4 mm. It was demonstrated in an elderly human model that a cylindrical bone plug improves fixation by 19.9% (845. 8 N versus 691.7 N) compared with a bone plug with a trapezoidal cross section. Although gap size was not measured, it will be smaller with a cylindrical bone plug than with a trapezoidal bone plug [33]. In what may be the best investigation of the topic using human and bovine tissue, the authors found that, although screw diameter or gap size alone was not significant, interference (defined as the screw's outer thread diameter minus the tunnel–bone block gap) was significantly related to load at failure in the pooled specimens and in the bovine model [15]. A number of authors have suggested using larger screws as the gap size increases [34].

Screw length probably does not have a large influence on the initial fixation properties of bone-patella tendon-bone grafts fixed with interference screws. Brown and colleagues [30] found no significant difference in fixation strength between 7 × 20-mm and 7 × 30-mm screws or between 9 × 20-mm and 9 × 30-mm screws fixed in the distal femur of human specimens. Black and colleagues [35] compared 9 × 12.5-mm, 9 × 15-mm, and 9 × 20-mm interference screws in a porcine tibia model. No significant differences in insertion torque, failure load, stiffness, or displacement to failure was found among the different-length screws. Pomeroy and colleagues [36] also found no significant effect of screw length on fixation strength for a given screw diameter. Fixation strength is not improved by using an interference screw longer than the bone plug.

Divergence of the interference screw from the bone block and the axis of the bone tunnel can occur with both rear-entry and endoscopic techniques. The incidence of screw divergence is more common with the endoscopic technique (femur > tibia) [37]. Using a porcine model, Jomha and colleagues [38] reported no significant difference in femoral fixation strength with endoscopically inserted interference screws with divergence up to 10°, but there was a significant decrease with screw divergence of 20° or greater. Pierz and colleagues [39], using porcine tibias, demonstrated that interference screws inserted to simulate a rear-entry femoral fixation technique or fixation of a tibial bone block resulted in a significant decrease in fixation strength with divergence between 0° and 15° compared with 15° to 30° of divergence. Interference screws inserted to simulate an endoscopic technique resulted in a significant decrease in fixation strength only at 30° of screw divergence. These authors concluded that optimal interference screw fixation occurs when the screw is placed parallel to the bone block and bone tunnel. Because of the creation of a wedge effect, screw divergence has less effect on endoscopically inserted femoral screws. Based on clinical studies, screw divergence of less than 30° does not seem to have a significant effect on the clinical outcome [40]. Because of the in-line direction of pull, however, minor degrees of divergence have a greater effect on the fixation strength of femoral screws inserted through a rear-entry technique and tibial fixation screws.

Metal interference screws can distort MRI images, lacerate the graft during insertion, and complicate revision ACL surgery. Bioabsorbable interference screws have been proposed as a method to eliminate potential complications [41]. Several biomechanical studies have compared the initial fixation strength of bioabsorbable interference screws and conventional metal interference screws in animal and human cadaveric models. These studies showed that most bioabsorbable interference screws provide fixation strength similar to that of metal interference screws and concluded that the use of these screws may allow an accelerated postoperative rehabilitation program [42–48].

Concerns with bioabsorbable interference screws have focused largely on the issues of screw breakage and biocompatibility. Screw breakage has been addressed largely by designing screws and screwdrivers that allow the insertion torque to be distributed along the entire length of the screw and by decreasing the insertion torque by notching the bone tunnel wall. To prevent screw breakage, it is important that the screwdriver be engaged fully during insertion of the screw.

In summary, based on a review of the literature, gap size is probably the most important factor influencing the initial fixation properties of interference screw fixation of bone-tendon-bone grafts. Gap size also is the one factor that can be measured easily intraoperatively and controlled by the surgeon. Improvements in initial graft fixation can be achieved by increasing the diameter of the screw to compensate for the gap size. Increasing screw length seems to offer minimal improvements in initial graft fixation properties.

Guidelines and Recommendations for Intratunnel Fixation of Bone-Tendon-Bone Grafts

Femoral fixation: two-incision technique

The authors recommend using metal screws 7 and 8 mm in diameter with a length of 20 to 25 mm. Bioabsorbable screws can be used, but the higher insertion torque generated by the insertion of the screw against the hard cortex of distal femur may result in a higher incidence of screw breakage compared with bioabsorbable screws inserted using an endoscopic technique. When the gap between the bone block and bone tunnel wall is greater than 4 mm, suture/post or plastic button fixation should be considered in addition to intratunnel fixation.

Femoral fixation: endoscopic technique

The authors recommend using metal or bioabsorbable screws 8 or 9 mm in diameter, with a length of 20 to 25 mm. For bioabsorbable screws, one should review and use the manufacturer's guidelines regarding tapping or notching the bone tunnel wall to minimize the risk of screw breakage. The authors prefer using the EndoButton CL (Closed Loop; Smith and Nephew, Andover, Massachusetts) to avoid graft–tunnel mismatch in long grafts when the gap size is greater than 4 mm and when blowout of the posterior wall of the femoral tunnel occurs.

Tibial fixation

The authors recommend using screws 8 or 9 mm in diameter with a length of 20 to 25 mm. For gap sizes greater than 4 mm, one should consider suture/post or button as hybrid fixation. In soft bone or when low insertion torque is encountered, one should consider backing up the interference screw fixation by tying sutures around a fixation post.

SOFT TISSUE GRAFTS

Interference screw fixation of soft tissue grafts depends on many of the same factors as fixation for bone-patella tendon-bone grafts; but the relative importance of each of these factors differs [49]. As in bone-tendon-bone grafts, the initial fixation properties depend on the fixation device generating friction between the soft tissue graft and the bone tunnel wall. Friction is generated by compression of the soft tissue graft against the bone tunnel wall. Because the soft tissue graft is more compressible than the bone blocks of bone-tendon-bone grafts, a screw of a given diameter generates compression between the screw and bone tunnel wall. The amount of friction contributed by engagement of the screw threads in the bone tunnel wall and soft tissue graft also is significantly lower because of the lack of engagement of the screw threads into the soft tissue graft. As illustrated in Fig. 2, factors that may contribute to the initial fixation properties of soft tissue grafts with interference screws are

1. Screw geometry (length and diameter)
2. Tendon fit
3. Tunnel impaction or dilation
4. Screw placement (concentric versus eccentric)

Unlike interference screw fixation of bone-tendon-bone grafts, screw length seems to have a greater effect on the initial fixation properties of soft tissue grafts fixed with interference screws. Because of the lower BMD of the proximal tibia, screw length has a greater influence on tibial fixation properties [27]. Screw length may have a more significant effect on the fixation properties of soft tissue grafts because the area over which friction is generated between

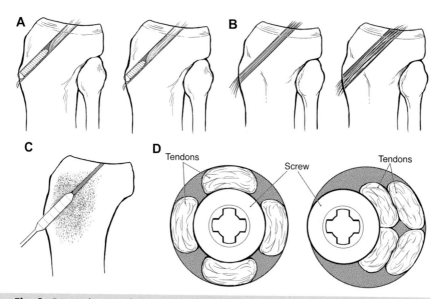

Fig. 2. Factors that contribute to the initial fixation properties of soft tissue grafts with interference screws. (A) Screw geometry (length and diameter): length and diameter of screw can affect construct strength. (B) Tendon fit: more precise fit to 0.5 mm allows improved strength with screw insertion. (C) Tunnel impaction or dilation: impaction drilling or serial dilation does not seem to significantly improve graft mechanics. (D) Screw placement (concentric versus eccentric): concentric or eccentric screw placement does not affect construct strength.

the bone tunnel wall and soft tissue graft is determined by the screw length, rather than by the length of a bone block, which is typically 20 to 25 mm. In a bovine proximal tibia model, Weiler and colleagues [50] found that 23-mm screws had lower pull-out strengths than 28-mm screws with equivalent diameters. This study also found that increasing screw length had a greater influence on failure load than increasing the screw diameter. Using human tibias (age range, 24–45 years), Selby and colleagues [51] demonstrated significantly higher ultimate failure loads for screws 35 mm long than for screws 28 mm long. Placing the screw so that it engaged the cortex of the tibia allowed significantly less slippage than screw insertion that engaged only cancellous bone [52]. Based on their findings, the authors recommend that the screw head be placed to engage the tibial cortex.

Few studies have examined the influence of screw diameter on the initial fixation properties of soft tissue ACL grafts fixed with interference screws. Using human hamstring tendons grafts and bovine proximal tibias, Weiler and colleagues [50] found that increasing the diameter of a 23-mm length bio-absorbable interference screw from 7 mm to 8 mm increased the mean pull-out force from 367 N to 479 N.

The fit of the soft tissue graft in the bone tunnel seems to have a significant influence on the initial fixation properties of interference screw fixation of soft tissue grafts. Using a human cadaveric model, Steenlage and colleagues [53] demonstrated that QHTGs fixed in the distal femur with a bioabsorbable screw had a significantly higher ultimate failure load if the bone tunnel was sized within 0.5 mm of the graft diameter rather than within 1 mm of the graft diameter.

Because BMD has such a significant effect on the initial tensile properties of interference screw fixation of soft tissue grafts, compaction drilling or bone tunnel dilation has been proposed as a method of creating increased bone density along the bone tunnel walls. It has been speculated that this approach will improve initial fixation properties. Using human male cadaveric knees, Rittmeister and colleagues [54] found that serial dilation failed to improve the initial fixation strength of QHTGs fixed in the tibia with metal interferences screws. Nurmi and colleagues [55] investigated the effects of compaction drilling versus conventional or extraction drilling on the initial fixation strength of QHTGs fixed with bioabsorbable screws in the proximal tibia of human specimens (mean age, 41 ± 11 years; range, 17–49 years). The biomechanical testing protocol consisted of cyclic loading followed by a single load-to-failure test. They found no significant difference in initial stiffness or displacement between the two drilling methods during cyclic testing or in the single load-to-failure test and detected no significant differences between the two drilling methods in yield load, displacement at yield load, or stiffness.

In a second biomechanical study, Nurmi and colleagues [56] investigated the effect of tunnel compaction by serial dilators compared with conventional drilling on the initial fixation strength of doubled anterior tibial tendons fixed in the proximal tibia of human specimens (mean age, 40 ± 11 years; range,

17–54 years) using bioabsorbable interference screws. The specimens were tested under cyclic loading followed by a single load-to-failure test. Although no significant difference in stiffness or displacement between the two techniques was demonstrated during cyclic testing, the number of failures during cyclic loading of the extraction drilling group was twice that of the serially dilated group. In the subsequent single load-to-failure test, there was no significant difference in failure load or stiffness between the two groups. A limitation of this study was the size of the tibial bone tunnel was not matched to the size of the soft tissue grafts: a bone tunnel 10 mm in diameter was created in all specimens.

The only study to demonstrate a beneficial effect of tunnel dilation on the fixation strength of soft tissue ACL grafts was performed by Cain and colleagues [57] using paired human cadaveric knees (average age, 42 years; range, 29–47 years). QHTGs were fixed with bioabsorbable screws in 0.5-mm size-matched femoral and tibial tunnels. The tibial tunnel was created using smooth tunnel dilators in one knee of the pair, and extraction drilling was used in the opposite knee of the pair. The femur-hamstring ACL graft-tibia complex was tested to failure using anterior tibial translation with the knee positioned in 20° of flexion, as previously described by Steiner and colleagues [3]. This method of testing attempts to mimic the Lachman test. All specimens failed by the graft pulling out of the tibial tunnel, but the ultimate failure load was significantly higher for the dilated tibial tunnels. Testing methodology makes it difficult to compare the results of this study with earlier studies; however, based on the literature, the benefits of compaction drilling or serial dilation probably do not justify the extra cost and operating time.

Although there is general agreement that interference screws should be inserted on the cancellous side of bone-tendon-bone grafts, controversy exists regarding placement of tibial interference screws used to fix multiple-stranded hamstring tendon grafts. Soft tissue grafts may be fixed by inserting the screw on the side (eccentrically) or down the center (concentrically) of the graft strands. Concentric screw placement maximizes contact between the graft strands and the bone tunnel wall, providing a greater surface area for healing. Simonian and colleagues [58] were unable to detect a significant difference in initial fixation properties between eccentric versus concentric interference screw position against a model of human hamstring tendon grafts fixed in a polyurethane foam. Shino and Pflaster [59] investigated the effect of eccentric versus concentric screw placement on the initial fixation properties of QHTGs fixed in the proximal tibia of paired human cadaveric knees (average age, 51 years; range, 49–54 years). There were no significant differences in stiffness, yield load, ultimate failure load, or slippage between the two screw positions.

As with bone-patellar tendon-bone grafts, QHTGs in elderly human bone tunnels, bioabsorbable interference screws provide initial biomechanical fixation properties similar to those of a metal interference screw [60]. In the laboratory, two separate investigations have noted an association between a metal interference screw applied against a soft tissue graft and graft laceration or damage. Brand and colleagues [60], using human QHTG in elderly cadaver bone, noted a greater rate of graft laceration in the group in which a metal screw was used than in the group in which a bioabsorbable screw of comparable dimensions was used. Another group compared the effect of a single insertion of a metal screw versus the use two separate bioabsorbable screws, a poly-D,L-lactide and a poly-D,L-lactide with tricalcium phosphate. After the screws had been inserted, the soft tissue grafts were tested to failure. The metal screw damaged the tendon more extensively, resulting in a significantly smaller load at failure and stiffness than seen in the tendons damaged by bioabsorbable screws [61].

Guidelines and Recommendations for Intratunnel Fixation of Soft Tissue Grafts

Unlike bone-tendon-bone grafts, in which the bone tunnel size and dimensions of the bone blocks are standardized, there are large variations in the diameter and length of soft tissue grafts. These variations make it difficult to arrive at definitive recommendations regarding selection of interference screw fixation. Nevertheless, the authors' interpretation of the literature has led to the following conclusions:

1. Because of the lower BMD, and because the line of applied force is parallel to the axis of the tibial tunnel, tibial fixation is weaker, less stiff, and more likely to slip under cyclic loading than fixation using the femoral fixation site.
2. Screw length has a more significant effect on the initial fixation properties of interference screw fixation of soft tissue ACL grafts than of bone-tendon-bone ACL grafts.
3. In biomechanical testing longer screws result in higher ultimate failure loads and stiffness and less slippage.
4. Fixation properties are improved by having the screw head engage the tibial cortex.
5. The effect of screw diameter on initial fixation properties is unclear, making it difficult to establish clear guidelines for screw sizing.
6. Matching the size of the bone tunnel to within 0.5 mm of the measured size of the graft may improve initial fixation properties.
7. Compaction drilling or serial dilation does not seem to improve initial fixation properties significantly.

ALTERNATIVE INTRATUNNEL TIBIAL FIXATION TECHNIQUES

The stimulus for the development of alternative intratunnel tibial fixation techniques for soft tissue ACL grafts arose from the desire to decrease slippage and the high rate of fixation failure reported with interference screws under cyclic loading conditions; to eliminate or reduce the need for supplemental tibial fixation; and to improve soft tissue-to-bone healing at the graft-fixation sites [49,52,62]. The IntraFix (DePuy Mitek, Norwood, Massachusetts) was designed to capture individually each of the four strands of a soft tissue graft in a separate compartment using a plastic sheath and to achieve direct compression of each of the graft strands against the bone tunnel wall by the insertion of a tapered screw into the central chamber of the plastic sheath [62]. In a porcine tibia model using human hamstring tendon grafts, Kousa and colleagues [63] demonstrated that the IntraFix had the highest load failure load (1309 $\pm$ 302 N) and stiffness (267 $\pm$ 36 N/mm) and the least amount of slippage (1.5 mm) after cyclic loading when compared with two cortical fixation techniques and three other interference screw fixation techniques. When used to fix a QHTG in a human tibial tunnel, the IntraFix device had a load at failure (796 $\pm$ 193 N versus 647 $\pm$ 269 N) and stiffness (49 $\pm$ 21.9 N/mm versus 64.5 $\pm$ 22 N/mm) similar to that of a bioabsorbable interference screw 35 mm in length [64].

The GTS System (Graft Tunnel Solution; Smith & Nephew Endoscopy, Andover, Massachusetts) is a intratunnel tibial fixation technique that positions a poly-L-lactic, tapered, fine-pitch screw concentrically within the four-strand soft tissue graft [65]. The screw features a tapered design and shorter thread distance, which enhances compression of the soft tissue graft in cancellous bone. The graft sleeve is a three-lumen, woven, nonabsorbable polypropylene mesh graft sleeve that organizes the four-strand soft tissue graft in the tibial tunnel. The graft sleeve prevents graft twisting during screw insertion, which helps maintain equal tension in the four graft strands, maximizes bone–tendon contact that enhances healing, and provides better compression of each ligament strand against the bone tunnel wall while protecting the graft strands from screw damage. Cyclic testing followed by single load-to-failure testing of the graft sleeve, tapered screw, and IntraFix has been performed using human doubled gracilis and semitendinosus tendon grafts in the proximal tibia of calf bone (2 years or younger) with BMD similar to that of the proximal tibia in young humans. There was no significant difference in slippage, ultimate failure load, or stiffness between the two devices.

HYBRID FIXATION

Although intratunnel fixation of soft tissue grafts has improved with longer tibial screws and precise sizing of grafts to tunnel diameters, concerns persist that initial fixation strength that is less than the strength of the native ACL bone construct allows graft-tunnel motion that may contribute to knee laxity. In particular, older women and other patients who have lower BMC are candidates for hybrid fixation that combines improved structural properties with the biomechanical and biologic advantages of joint-line interference-fit fixation to augment intratunnel devices [66]. The EndoPearl (Linvatec, Largo, Forida) linked with #5 Ethibond sutures (Ethicon, Somerville, New Jersey) against the tip of a bioabsorbable interference screw significantly improved femoral fixation when compared with a bioabsorbable interference screw in a femoral tunnel of a calf model as measured by maximum load-to-failure (658.9 $\pm$ 118.1 N versus 385.9 $\pm$ 185.6 N) and stiffness (41.7 $\pm$ 11 N/mm versus 25.7 $\pm$ 8.5 N/mm) [67]. Hammond and colleagues [66] evaluated femoral fixation of quadrupled flexor tendons in porcine bone using a bioabsorbable screw, EndoButton

CL, and hybrid fixation using an EndoButton CL and bioabsorbable screw. The hybrid fixation group demonstrated greater yield and ultimate failure loads and greater stiffness under displacement-controlled cyclic loads. In a similar study, Oh and colleagues [68] demonstrated that the addition of an interference screw to suspensory fixation using an EndoButton CL increased ultimate failure load and stiffness and decreased slippage. Although hybrid fixation has improved initial graft-fixation tensile properties in biomechanical studies, there have been no clinical studies demonstrating that it results in improved clinical results.

CLINICAL STUDIES

Ma and colleagues [69] compared fixation techniques with patients reconstructed with QHTG in a prospective, nonrandomized study. Fifteen patients in each group were fixed with either a bioabsorbable interference screw in the femoral or tibial bone tunnel or femoral fixation with an EndoButton and tibial fixation with a screw post. There were no significant differences in International Knee Documentation Committee (IKDC) knee scores (85 ± 11 versus 81 ± 17) or side-to-side KT differences (3.2 ± 2.6 mm versus 2.4 ± 1.8 mm). There was more tunnel widening (as measured in the femoral tunnel in the sagittal plane) in the group of patients in which the bioabsorbable screw was used than in the group of patients fixed with extracortical fixation. All other measurements of tunnel width were not significantly different between groups [69]. A prospective, nonrandomized clinical trial of patients who had QHTGs and bone-patellar tendon-bone grafts fixed with metal interference screws with a 5-year follow-up found only that the bone-patellar tendon-bone group had a greater rate of arthritis. There were no significant differences in KT 2000 maximum manual testing, the percentage of patients who had a normal Lachman's test, the number of patients who had an A or B IKDC knee score, or the return to level I or II activities (Table 2) [70]. The same group of patients was followed up again at a mean of 7 years postoperatively. There was a greater rate of arthritis on radiographic review by the IKDC criteria in the bone-patellar tendon-bone group (45%) than in the QHTG group (14%). The number of patients in the bone-patellar tendon-bone group with loss of extension increased significantly between the 5-year and 7-year follow-ups, but there was not a significant difference between the bone-patellar tendon-bone and QHTG groups in the number of patients who had extension loss (see Table 2) [71]. A prospective, randomized investigation from Slovenia compared 64 patients randomly assigned to receive bone-patellar tendon-bone grafts or QHTGs. Interference fixation was provided with a metal screw in the femoral socket and a bioabsorbable screw of similar dimensions in the tibial tunnel. These investigators also found a greater rate of arthritis in the bone-patellar tendon-bone group: 50% had at least grade B arthritis by the IKDC scoring sheet, compared with 17% in the QHTG group. There were no differences in KT 2000 maximum manual testing, the percentage of patients

Table 2

Clinical studies comparing quadrupled hamstring tendon grafts (QHTG) and bone-patella tendon-bone (BPTB) grafts, each fixed with interference fixation of both the tibial and femoral portions of the graft

Graft	KT 2000[a] < 3 mm	Normal Lachman's Test	IKDC A or B Knee	Graft Rupture[b]	Return to Activities	Comments
QHTG [70]	72	84	89	7/90	60 (Level I or II)	5-year follow-up with metal interference screw
BPTB [70]	82	90	90	3/90	69 (Level I or II)	5-year follow-up with metal interference screw
QHTG [71]	80	82	89	9/61	55 (Level I or II)	7-year follow-up with metal interference screw
BPTB [71]	74	76	85	4/59	52 (Level I or II)	7-year follow-up with metal interference screw
QHTG [72]	85	79	97	1/28	82 (Preinjury level)	5-year follow-up with metal screw in femur and bioabsorbable screw in tibia
BPTB [72]	81	85	97	1/26	88 (Preinjury level)	5-year follow-up with metal screw in femur and bioabsorbable screw in tibia

Abbreviation: IKDC, International Knee Documentation Committee.

[a] KT 2000, Lachman's test, and IKDC results are expressed as a percentage of the total number of patients in that group.

[b] Graft ruptures are the number patients with graft rupture as a numerator and the number of patients in each group as the denominator.

who had a normal Lachman's test, the number of patients who had an A or B IKDC knee score, or return to preinjury activities (see Table 2) [72].

FUTURE DIRECTIONS

The ideal ACL graft-fixation method would provide immediate rigid fixation that is strong enough, stiff enough, and able to resist slippage so that permanent elongation does not develop with the stresses of rehabilitation and activities of daily living. The fixation method should be low profile and should not require later removal because of local irritation and pain. Ideally, the device should be replaced by cancellous bone and result in the development of a normal histologic ligament-to-bone attachment site.

Future improvements in intratunnel ACL graft fixation will depend on better understanding of the in vivo forces experienced by the ACL with rehabilitation exercises and activities in the early postoperative period and of the biology of fixation-site healing. Osteoconductive or osteoinductive materials that will stimulate the development of normal osseous tissue are under development currently. Bone cement that will provide immediate rigid fixation and eventually be replaced by bone may be developed. On-going basic science research is directed at promoting and accelerating healing of soft tissue to bone. Ultrasound, bone morphogenetic proteins, and biologic growth factors currently are being investigated as possible methods to promote and accelerate tendon-to-bone healing.

References

[1] Lambert K. Vascularized patellar tendon graft with rigid internal fixation for anterior cruciate ligament insufficiency. Clin Orthop Relat Res 1983;172:85–9.

[2] Kurosaka M, Yoshiya S, Andrish J. A biomechanical comparison of different surgical techniques of graft fixation of anterior cruciate ligament reconstruction. Am J Sports Med 1987;15(3):225–9.

[3] Steiner M, Hecker A, Brown C. Anterior cruciate ligament graft fixation: comparison of hamstring and patellar tendon grafts. Am J Sports Med 1994;22(2):240–7.

[4] Bach B, Tradonsky S, Bojchuk J, et al. Arthroscopically assisted anterior cruciate ligament reconstruction using patellar tendon autograft. Five-to nine-year follow-up evaluation. Am J Sports Med 1998;26(1):20–9.

[5] Pinczewski L. Endoscopic ACL reconstruction utilizing a quadrupled hamstring tendon autograft with direct RCI interference screw fixation. Presented at the Lecture/Laboratory Session of RCI Screw, Smith & Nephew Donjoy. Columbus (GA), February, 1996.

[6] Fu F. Using bioabsorbable interference screw fixation for hamstring ACL-reconstruction. Orthopaedics Today 1997;16:36–7.

[7] Morrison J. Function of the knee joint in various activities. Biomed Eng 1969;4(12):573–80.

[8] Morrison J. The mechanics of the knee joint in relation to normal walking. J Biomech 1970;3:51–61.

[9] Noyes F, Butler D, Grood E, et al. Biomechanical analysis of human ligament grafts used in knee-ligament repairs and reconstructions. J Bone Joint Surg 1984;66(3):344–52.

[10] Cooper D, Deng X, Burstein A, et al. The strength of the central third patellar tendon graft: a biomechanical study. Am J Sports Med 1993;21(6):818–24.

[11] Hamner D, Brown C, Steiner M, et al. Hamstring tendon grafts for reconstruction of the anterior cruciate ligament: biomechanical evaluation of the use of multiple strands and tensioning techniques. J Bone Joint Surg Am 1999;81(4):549–57.

[12] Brand J, Weiler A, Caborn D, et al. Graft fixation in cruciate ligament reconstruction. Current concepts. Am J Sports Med 2000;28(5):764–74.

[13] Beynnon B, Amis A. In vitro testing protocols for cruciate ligaments and ligament reconstructions. Knee Surg Sports Traumatol Arthrosc 1998;6(Suppl 1):S70–6.

[14] Weiss J, Paulos L. Mechanical testing of ligament fixation devices. Techniques in Orthopaedics 1999;14:14–21.

[15] Brown G, Pena F, Grontvedt T, et al. Fixation strength of interference screw fixation in bovine, young human, and elderly human cadaver knees: influence of insertion torque, tunnel-bone block gap, and interference. Knee Surg Sports Traumatol Arthrosc 1996;3(4):238–44.

[16] Aerssens J, Boonen S, Lowet G, et al. Interspecies differences in bone composition, density, and quality: potential implications for in vivo bone research. Endocrinology 1998;139(2): 663–70.

[17] Nagarkatti D, McKeon B, Donahue B, et al. Mechanical evaluation of a soft tissue interference screw in free tendon anterior cruciate ligament graft fixation. Am J Sports Med 2001;29(1):67–71.

[18] Nurmi J, Sievanen H, Kannus P, et al. Porcine tibia is a poor substitute for human cadaver tibia for evaluating interference screw fixation. Am J Sports Med 2004;32(3):765–71.

[19] Shapiro J, Jackson D, Aberman H, et al. Comparison of pullout strength for seven- and nine-millimeter diameter interference screw size as used in anterior cruciate ligament reconstruction. Arthroscopy 1995;11(5):596–9.

[20] Bryan J, Bach B, Bush-Joseph C, et al. Comparison of "inside-out" and "outside-in" interference screw fixation for anterior cruciate ligament surgery in a bovine knee. Arthroscopy 1996;12(1):76–81.

[21] Hulstyn M, Fadale P, Abate J, et al. Biomechanical evaluation of interference screw fixation in a bovine patellar bone-tendon-bone autograft complex for anterior cruciate ligament reconstruction. Arthroscopy 1993;9(4):417–24.

[22] Clancy W, Narechania R, Rosenberg T, et al. Anterior and posterior cruciate ligament reconstruction in Rhesus monkeys. A histological microangiographic and biomechanical analysis. J Bone Joint Surg 1981;63(8):1270–84.

[23] Walton M. Absorbable and metal interference screws: comparison of graft security during healing. Arthroscopy 1999;15(8):818–26.

[24] Rodeo S, Arnoczky S, Torzilli P, et al. Tendon healing in a bone tunnel. J Bone Joint Surg 1993;75(12):1795–803.

[25] Milano G, Mulas P, Sanna-Passino E, et al. Evaluation of bone plug and soft tissue anterior cruciate ligament graft fixation over time using transverse femoral fixation in a sheep model. Arthroscopy 2005;21(5):532–9.

[26] Cassim A, Lobenhoffer P, Gerich T. The fixation strength of the interference screw in anterior cruciate ligament replacement as a function of technique and experimental setup. Transactions Orthopaedic Research Society 1993;18:31.

[27] Brand J, Pienkowski D, Steenlage E, et al. Interference screw fixation strength of quadrupled hamstring tendon graft is directly related to bone mineral density and insertion torque. Am J Sports Med 2000;28(5):705–10.

[28] Jarvinen M, Nurmi J, Sievanen H. Bone density and insertion torque as predictors of anterior cruciate ligament graft fixation strength. Am J Sports Med 2004;32(6):1421–9.

[29] Kohn D, Rose C. Primary stability of interference screw fixation: influence of screw diameter and insertion torque. Am J Sports Med 1994;22(3):334–8.

[30] Brown C, Hecker A, Hipp J. The biomechanics of interference screw fixation of patellar tendon anterior cruciate ligament grafts. Am J Sports Med 1993;21(6):880–6.

[31] Butler J, Branch T, Hutton W. Optimal graft fixation-the effect of gap size and screw size on bone plug fixation in ACL reconstruction. Arthroscopy 1994;10(5):524–9.

[32] Reznik A, Davis J, Daniel D. Optimizing interference fixation for cruciate ligament reconstruction. Transactions Orthopaedic Research Society 1990;15:519.

[33] Shapiro J, Cohn B, Jackson D, et al. The biomechanical effects of geometric configuration of bone-tendon-bone autografts in anterior cruciate ligament reconstruction. Arthroscopy 1992;8(4):453–8.

[34] Fithian D, Daniel D, Casanave A. Fixation in knee ligament repair and reconstruction. Operative Techniques in Orthopaedics 1992;2:63–70.

[35] Black K, Saunders M, Stube K, et al. Effects of interference fit screw length on tibial tunnel fixation for anterior cruciate ligament reconstruction. Am J Sports Med 2000;28(6):846–9.

[36] Pomeroy G, Baltz M, Pierz K, et al. The effects of bone plug length and screw diameter on the holding strength of bone-tendon-bone grafts. Arthroscopy 1998;14(2):148–52.

[37] Lemos M, Albert J, Simon T, et al. Radiographic analysis of femoral interference screw placement during ACL reconstruction: endoscopic versus open technique. Arthroscopy 1993;9(2):154–8.

[38] Jomha N, Raso V, Leung P. Effect of varying angles on the pullout strength of interference screw fixation. Arthroscopy 1993;9(5):580–3.

[39] Pierz K, Baltz M, Fulkerson J. The effect of Kurosaka screw divergence on the holding strength of bone-tendon-bone grafts. Am J Sports Med 1995;23(3):332–5.

[40] Dworsky B, Jewell B, Bach B. Interference screw divergence in endoscopic anterior cruciate ligament reconstruction. Arthroscopy 1996;12(1):45–9.

[41] Barber F, Elrod B, McGuire D, et al. Preliminary results of an absorbable interference screw. Arthroscopy 1995;11(5):537–48.

[42] Weiler A, Windhagen H, Raschke M, et al. Biodegradable interference screw fixation exhibits pull-out force and stiffness similar to titanium screws. Am J Sports Med 1998;26(1): 119–28.

[43] Kousa P, Jarvinen T, Kannus P, et al. Initial fixation strength of bioabsorbable and titanium interference screws in anterior cruciate ligament reconstruction: biomechanical evaluation by single cycle and cyclic loading. Am J Sports Med 2001;29(4):420–5.

[44] Johnson L, vanDyk G. Metal and biodegradable interference screws: comparison of failure strength. Arthroscopy 1996;12(4):452–6.

[45] Caborn D, Urban W, Johnson D, et al. Biomechanical comparison between bioscrew and titanium alloy interference screws for bone-patellar tendon-bone graft fixation in anterior cruciate ligament reconstruction. Arthroscopy 1997;13(2):229–32.

[46] Abate J, Fadale P, Hulstyn M, et al. Initial fixation strength of polylactic acid interference screws in anterior cruciate ligament reconstruction. Arthroscopy 1998;14(3):278–84.

[47] Pena F, Grontvedt T, Brown G, et al. Comparison of failure strength between metallic and absorbable interference screws. Influence of insertion torque, tunnel-bone block gap, bone mineral density, and interference. Am J Sports Med 1996;24(3):329–34.

[48] Rupp S, Krauss P, Fritsch E. Fixation strength of a biodegradable interference screw and a press-fit technique in anterior cruciate ligament reconstruction with a BPTB graft. Arthroscopy 1997;13(1):61–5.

[49] Brand J, Caborn D, Johnson D. Biomechanics of soft tissue interference screw fixation for anterior cruciate ligament reconstruction. Orthopedics 2003;26(4):432–9.

[50] Weiler A, Hoffman R, Siepe C, et al. The influence of screw geometry on hamstring tendon interference fit fixation. Am J Sports Med 2000;28(3):356–9.

[51] Selby J, Johnson D, Hester P, et al. Effect of screw length on bioabsorbable interference screw fixation in a tibial bone tunnel. Am J Sports Med 2000;29(5):614–9.

[52] Harvey A, Thomas N, Amis A. The effect of screw length and position on fixation of four-stranded hamstring grafts for anterior cruciate ligament reconstruction. Knee 2003;10(1):97–102.

[53] Steenlage E, Brand J, Johnson D, et al. Correlation of bone tunnel diameter with quadrupled hamstring strength using a biodegradable interference screw. Arthroscopy 2002;18(8): 901–7.

[54] Rittmeister M, Noble P, Bocell J, et al. Interactive effects of tunnel dilation on the mechanical properties of hamstring grafts fixed in the tibia with interference screws. Knee Surg Sports Traumatol Arthrosc 2001;9(5):267–71.

[55] Nurmi J, Kannus P, Sievanen H, et al. Compaction drilling does not increase the initial fixation strength of the hamstring tendon graft in anterior cruciate ligament reconstruction in a cadaver model. Am J Sports Med 2003;31(3):353–8.

[56] Nurmi J, Kannus P, Sievanen H, et al. Interference screw fixation of soft tissue grafts in anterior cruciate ligament reconstruction: part 1. Effect of tunnel compaction by serial dilators versus extraction drilling on the initial fixation strength. Am J Sports Med 2004;32(2): 411–7.

[57] Cain E, Phillips B, Charlebois S, et al. Effect of tibial tunnel dilation on pullout strength of semitendinosus-gracilis graft in anterior cruciate ligament reconstruction. Orthopedics 2005;28(8):779–83.

[58] Simonian P, Sussman P, Baldini T. Interference screw position and hamstring graft location for ACL reconstruction. Presented at the 17th Annual Meeting of Arthroscopy Association of North America. Orlando (FL), April 30–May 3, 1998.

[59] Shino K, Pflaster D. Comparison of eccentric and concentric screw placement for hamstring graft fixation in the tibial tunnel. Knee Surg Sports Traumatol Arthrosc 2000;8(2):73–5.

[60] Brand J, Nyland J, Caborn D, et al. Soft-tissue interference fixation: bioabsorbable screw versus metal screw. Arthroscopy 2005;21(8):911–6.

[61] Zantop T, Weimann A, Schmidtko R, et al. Graft laceration and pullout strength of soft-tissue anterior cruciate ligament reconstruction: in vitro study comparing titanium, poly-D,L-lactide, and poly-D,L-lactide-tricalcium phosphate screws. Arthroscopy 2006;22(11):1204–10.

[62] Magen H, Howell S, Hull M. Structural properties of six tibial fixation methods for anterior cruciate ligament soft tissue grafts. Am J Sports Med 1999;27(1):35–43.

[63] Kousa P, Jarvinen T, Vihavainen M, et al. The fixation strength of six hamstring tendon graft fixation devices in anterior cruciate ligament reconstruction. Part II: tibial site. Am J Sports Med 2003;31(2):182–8.

[64] Caborn D, Brand J, Nyland J, et al. A biomechanical comparison of initial soft tissue fixation devices: the Intrafix versus a tapered 35-mm bioabsorbable interference screw. Am J Sports Med 2004;32(4):956–61.

[65] Brown C, Darwich N. Anterior cruciate ligament reconstruction using autogenous doubled gracilis and semitendinosus tendons with GTS sleeve and tapered screw fixation. Techniques in Orthopaedics 2005;20:290–6.

[66] Hammond G, Armstrong K, McGarry M, et al. Hybrid fixation improves structural properties of a free tendon anterior cruciate ligament reconstruction. Arthroscopy 2006;22(7):781–6.

[67] Weiler A, Richter M, Schmidmaier G, et al. The EndoPearl device increases fixation strength and eliminates construct slippage of hamstring tendon grafts with interference screw fixation. Arthroscopy 2001;17(4):353–9.

[68] Oh Y, Namkoong S, Strauss E, et al. Hybrid femoral fixation of soft-tissue grafts in anterior cruciate ligament reconstruction using EndoButton CL and bioabsorbable interference screws: a biomechanical study. Arthroscopy 2006;22(11):1218–24.

[69] Ma C, Francis K, Towers J, et al. Hamstring anterior cruciate ligament reconstruction: A comparison of bioabsorbable interference screw and EndoButton-post fixation. Arthroscopy 2004;20(2):122–8.

[70] Pinczewski L, Deehan D, Salmon L, et al. A five-year comparison of patellar tendon versus four-strand hamstring tendon autograft for arthroscopic reconstruction of the anterior cruciate ligament. Am J Sports Med 2002;30(4):523–36.

[71] Roe J, Pinczewski L, Russell V, et al. A 7-year follow-up of patellar tendon and hamstring tendon grafts for arthroscopic anterior cruciate ligament reconstruction. Am J Sports Med 2005;33:1337–45.

[72] Sajovic M, Vengust V, Komadina R, et al. A prospective, randomized comparison of semitendinosus and gracilis tendon versus patellar tendon autografts for anterior cruciate ligament reconstruction. Am J Sports Med 2006;34(12):1933–40.

INDEX

A

Note: Page numbers of article titles are in **boldface** type.

0278-5919/07/$ – see front matter
doi:10.1016/S0278-5919(07)00083-X

United States Postal Service

Statement of Ownership, Management, and Circulation
(All Periodicals Publications Except Requestor Publications)

1. Publication Title	2. Publication Number								3. Filing Date
Clinics in Sports Medicine	0	0	0	-	7	0	2		9/14/07

4. Issue Frequency	5. Number of Issues Published Annually	6. Annual Subscription Price
Jan, Apr, Jul, Oct	4	$205.00

7. Complete Mailing Address of Known Office of Publication (Not printer) (Street, city, county, state, and ZIP+4)

Elsevier Inc.
360 Park Avenue South
New York, NY 10010-1710

Contact Person
Stephen Bushing

Telephone (Include area code)
215-239-3688

8. Complete Mailing Address of Headquarters or General Business Office of Publisher (Not printer)

Elsevier Inc., 360 Park Avenue South, New York, NY 10010-1710

9. Full Names and Complete Mailing Addresses of Publisher, Editor, and Managing Editor (Do not leave blank)

Publisher (Name and complete mailing address)

John Schrefer - Elsevier, Inc., 1600 John F. Kennedy Blvd. Suite 1800, Philadelphia, PA 19103-2899

Editor (Name and complete mailing address)

Deb Dellapena, Elsevier, Inc., 1600 John F. Kennedy Blvd. Suite 1800, Philadelphia, PA 19103-2899

Managing Editor (Name and complete mailing address)

Catherine Bewick, Elsevier, Inc., 1600 John F. Kennedy Blvd. Suite 1800, Philadelphia, PA 19103-2899

10. Owner (Do not leave blank. If the publication is owned by a corporation, give the name and address of the corporation immediately followed by the names and addresses of all stockholders owning or holding 1 percent or more of the total amount of stock. If not owned by a corporation, give the names and addresses of the individual owners. If owned by a partnership or other unincorporated firm, give its name and address as well as those of each individual owner. If the publication is published by a nonprofit organization, give its name and address.)

Full Name	Complete Mailing Address
Wholly owned subsidiary of	4520 East-West Highway
Reed/Elsevier, US holdings	Bethesda, MD 20814

11. Known Bondholders, Mortgagees, and Other Security Holders Owning or Holding 1 Percent or More of Total Amount of Bonds, Mortgages, or Other Securities. If none, check box ☐ None

Full Name	Complete Mailing Address
N/A	

12. Tax Status (For completion by nonprofit organizations authorized to mail at nonprofit rates) (Check one)
The purpose, function, and nonprofit status of this organization and the exempt status for federal income tax purposes:
☐ Has Not Changed During Preceding 12 Months
☐ Has Changed During Preceding 12 Months (Publisher must submit explanation of change with this statement)

PS Form 3526, September 2006 (Page 1 of 3 (Instructions Page 3)) PSN 7530-01-000-9931 PRIVACY NOTICE: See our Privacy policy in www.usps.com

13. Publication Title	14. Issue Date for Circulation Data Below
Clinics in Sports Medicine	April 2007

15. Extent and Nature of Circulation			14. Average No. Copies Each Issue During Preceding 12 Months	No. Copies of Single Issue Published Nearest to Filing Date
a. Total Number of Copies (Net press run)			2200	2100
b. Paid Circulation (By Mail and Outside the Mail)	(1)	Mailed Outside-County Paid Subscriptions Stated on PS Form 3541 (Include paid distribution above nominal rate, advertiser's proof copies, and exchange copies)	1294	1218
	(2)	Mailed In-County Paid Subscriptions Stated on PS Form 3541 (Include paid distribution above nominal rate, advertiser's proof copies, and exchange copies)		
	(3)	Paid Distribution Outside the Mails Including Sales Through Dealers and Carriers, Street Vendors, Counter Sales, and Other Paid Distribution Outside USPS®	280	271
	(4)	Paid Distribution by Other Classes Mailed Through the USPS (e.g. First-Class Mail®)		
c. Total Paid Distribution (Sum of 15b (1), (2), (3), and (4))			1574	1489
d. Free or Nominal Rate Distribution (By Mail and Outside the Mail)	(1)	Free or Nominal Rate Outside-County Copies included on PS Form 3541	123	90
	(2)	Free or Nominal Rate In-County Copies Included on PS Form 3541		
	(3)	Free or Nominal Rate Copies Mailed at Other Classes Mailed Through the USPS (e.g. First-Class Mail)		
	(4)	Free or Nominal Rate Distribution Outside the Mail (Carriers or other means)	123	90
e. Total Free or Nominal Rate Distribution (Sum of 15d (1), (2), (3) and (4))			123	90
f. Total Distribution (Sum of 15c and 15e)			1697	1579
g. Copies not Distributed (See instructions to publishers #4 (page #3))			503	521
h. Total (Sum of 15f and g)			2200	2100
i. Percent Paid (15c divided by 15f times 100)			92.75%	94.30%

16. Publication of Statement of Ownership

☑ If the publication is a general publication, publication of this statement is required. Will be printed ☐ Publication not required
in the October 2007 issue of this publication.

17. Signature and Title of Editor, Publisher, Business Manager, or Owner

[signature]

Stephen Bushing - Executive Director of Subscription Services

	Date
	September 14, 2007

I certify that all information furnished on this form is true and complete. I understand that anyone who furnishes false or misleading information on this form or who omits material or information requested on the form may be subject to criminal sanctions (including fines and imprisonment) and/or civil sanctions (including civil penalties).

PS Form 3526, September 2006 (Page 2 of 3)

Moving?

Make sure your subscription moves with you!

To notify us of your new address, find your **Clinics Account Number** (located on your mailing label above your name), and contact customer service at:

E-mail: elspcs@elsevier.com

800-654-2452 (subscribers in the U.S. & Canada)
407-345-4000 (subscribers outside of the U.S. & Canada)

Fax number: 407-363-9661

Elsevier Periodicals Customer Service
6277 Sea Harbor Drive
Orlando, FL 32887-4800

*To ensure uninterrupted delivery of your subscription, please notify us at least 4 weeks in advance of move.